CW01066609

Learning to care
in the
A & E DEPARTMENT

Gary J Jones
SRN, OND, DipN(Lond), REMT, FETC

Nursing Officer, Accident & Emergency Department, Orsett
Hospital, Grays, Essex

HODDER AND STOUGHTON
LONDON SYDNEY AUCKLAND TORONTO

LEARNING TO CARE SERIES

General Editors

JEAN HEATH, MEd, BA, SRN, SCM
English National Board Learning Resources Unit,
Sheffield

SUSAN E NORMAN, SRN, DNCERT, RNT
Senior Tutor, The Nightingale School, West Lambeth Health Authority

Titles in this series include:

Learning to Care for Elderly People
L THOMAS
Learning to Care in the Community
P TURTON and J ORR
Learning to Care on the Medical Ward
A MATTHEWS
Learning to Care on the ENT Ward
D STOKES
Learning to Care on the Gynaecology Ward
W SIMONS
Learning to Care on the Psychiatric Ward
M WARD
Learning to Care for Mentally Handicapped People
V POUNDS
Learning to Care on the Orthopaedic Ward
D JULIEN

British Library Cataloguing in Publication Data

Jones, Gary J.
   Learning to care in the A & E department.
   – (Learning to care series)
   1. Emergency nursing
   I. Title   II. Series
   610.73'61   RT120.E4

ISBN 0 340 29414 5

First published 1986
Copyright © 1986 Gary J Jones

Typeset in 10/11 pt Trump Mediaeval by Rowland Phototypesetting Ltd, Bury St Edmunds, Suffolk

Printed in Great Britain for Hodder and Stoughton Educational, a division of Hodder and Stoughton Ltd, Mill Road, Dunton Green, Sevenoaks, Kent TN13 2YD, by Richard Clay (The Chaucer Press) Ltd, Bungay, Suffolk

EDITORS' FOREWORD

In most professions there is a traditional gulf between theory and its practice, and nursing is no exception. The gulf is perpetuated when theory is taught in a theoretical setting and practice is taught by the practitioner.

This inherent gulf has to be bridged by students of nursing, and publication of this series is an attempt to aid such bridge building.

It aims to help relate theory and practice in a meaningful way whilst underlining the importance of the person being cared for.

It aims to introduce students of nursing to some of the more common problems found in each new area of experience in which they will be asked to work.

It aims to de-mystify some of the technical language they will hear, putting it in context, giving it meaning and enabling understanding.

PREFACE

Nursing care within the Accident & Emergency department is as exciting and diverse as the patients coming through the department any day. This field of nursing is totally different to ward care; patients spend less time with the nurse and it is important to gain the patients' trust in this short period. The aim of this book is to provide the learner with a basic introduction to nursing within the Accident & Emergency department.

Using the Nursing Process system for planning care, the book has approached the subject with the thought in mind that not all nurses will be able to follow through a given patient from arrival until discharge or admission to the ward. Nurses may interact with a patient during any of the Assessment, Implementation or Evaluation stages of care. It may only be possible in some circumstances for nurses to meet patients at the admission or discharge stage of their care. For this reason the book includes the care in the Accident & Emergency department during all of these stages, so that the nurse may refer to individual chapters if dealing with patients at any one particular stage in the total care of the individual.

The book has deliberately avoided in-depth detail of practical skills such as various bandaging or specific techniques; what it does provide is a broad framework on which to build your knowledge.

Some repetition between chapters has intentionally been included; this allows the nurse the convenience of not turning to other chapters when dealing with a specific area of care.

CONTENTS

Introduction

Welcome to Accident & Emergency nursing, possibly the most diverse, yet interesting, area of your training. At present you will be very unsure of your role in this area of patient care.

You may well already be anxious about your allocation, imagining every patient arriving with severe injuries or illness. Yes, of course, patients come with life threatening conditions, but by far the majority of your patients will have minor injuries or illness and be quite able to return home after treatment. Why then, you may ask, if the majority of Accident & Emergency patients have minor injuries, do we need such a dramatic title as Accident & Emergency? Why not remain with the familiar word Casualty?

In 1962 the Platt Report on Accident & Emergency services in the NHS recommended a reduction in what is termed 'Casual Attenders' or patients who could have attended their GP. In fact, the Platt Report led directly to the redesignation of Casualty departments to Accident & Emergency departments. This change of name has not, however, changed the use of the department. In 1983 eleven London Accident & Emergency departments estimated that 50 per cent of patients did not fall within the classification of requiring hospital treatment. You will see during your allocation that many patients appear not to warrant Accident & Emergency care; however, as a nurse allocated to the department, all patients, irrespective of their condition and needs, must be treated in the most courteous and professional manner. It is our job to provide high quality nursing care, not to judge a person's use or misuse of this department.

During your allocation you must always remember that the Accident & Emergency department is the 'shop window' of any hospital. The care we give, and the attitude we portray, will affect many people. Often the only perception people have of a hospital is from the Accident & Emergency department.

Nursing in Accident & Emergency

The first point of the Code of Nursing ethics of the International Council of Nurses states:

1 The fundamental responsibility of the nurse is threefold – *to conserve life, alleviate suffering* and *to promote health*.

The nurse in Accident & Emergency has the opportunity to fulfill all three. Each day will hold a new challenge, a person in need. Nursing here requires an open mind and the ability to respond to the situation at hand. The nurse must be prepared to challenge existing procedures and provide the most modern and skilled care available. As a nurse learner you will be expected to deal with all manner of patients and conditions, from a cut finger to a cardiac arrest, from the suicidal patient to the elderly lady worried about her arthritis. You will not have to deal with all of these alone, there is always trained staff on duty. Always observe the trained staff at work and question their methods in order to develop your own Accident & Emergency nursing skills.

To Conserve Life

A small percentage of patients seen in the Accident & Emergency department require life saving skills such as cardiac and respiratory resuscitation. Conserving life however

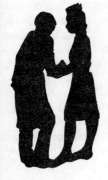

must not be viewed entirely around this type of care. A patient severely depressed, possibly having taken an overdose of drugs, may not be at risk from death due to his action. His life however may be severely affected – life is not just a case of living or dying, the quality of it is important. The elderly man who has lost his wife may cry on your shoulder, saying his life is over, he cannot go on without his wife after 50 years together. A gentle word, a caring approach, a smile at the right moment, may be the help he requires; you may conserve his life in this way. In the Accident & Emergency department you will have the opportunity of seeing and being involved in both types of life preservation, but always remember, quality as well as quantity of years is important.

Alleviate Suffering

All patients are suffering in some way when they arrive at an Accident & Emergency department. Pain is a major contribution to suffering. Analgesics can be prescribed by the medical staff, but much alleviation of suffering can be achieved by correct nursing care, such as proper support of fractured limbs, correct movement of patients with spinal injury, and correct positioning of patients with respiratory difficulty. However minor a patient's injury or illness, there will always be stress suffered by that person. A calm and orderly approach by nursing staff, accompanied by a friendly welcome and reassurance will do much to relieve this anxiety.

Promote Health

This is a large part of nursing care that can be practised by nurses in Accident & Emergency. Health education is the key to good health and often nursing staff have the opportunity to promote this when the patient is in the department. Explanation of cross infection, care of

A febrile convulsion is a period of spasmodic contraction of muscles due to a high temperature in the young child. Often referred to as a 'fit'

Conjunctivitis is inflammation of the conjunctiva, usually caused by bacteria or virus

Debridement is surgical removal of injured tissue and foreign bodies from a contaminated wound.

wounds, the necessity of locking medication away from children, how to prevent febrile convulsions in your child, are all possible examples of the nurse promoting health in the community.

The person suffering conjunctivitis of one eye will have an explanation given on cross infection. The towel he has used can infect his other eye or those of other family members, as can touching the eye and directly transferring the bacteria in that manner.

Correct care of frozen food may prevent a future visit after a complaint of abdominal pain, diarrhoea and vomiting.

Promoting health is a major part of patient care and will often determine the outcome of patients' treatment. An example of this is a patient with a burn to the arm. The burn is examined by the doctor, the depth and extent of burn determined and treatment prescribed. The treatment will usually take the form of cleaning the burn, removing dead tissue and application of a dressing. This will all be undertaken by the nurse. Subsequent dressings, debridement and care will also be dealt with by the nurse in a Follow-Up Clinic within the department. Thus, it is evident that the correct nursing care undertaken is the major part of that patient's treatment and subsequent well being. At any time incorrect application of that skill could result in infection (often long term), scarring (more than necessary) and long term effects to the patient, both physically and psychologically.

The incorrectly applied bandage can be as detrimental to a patient's health and recovery as can the incorrect handling of a person with spinal injury. Always remember one golden rule – if in doubt, ask. Never be afraid to admit you are not sure. Remember as most patients go home, if your care has been incorrect, no one can reverse it.

Methods will vary

So many times learners express their concern about practical procedures where one trained nurse has shown one method and another nurse a variation on that method. Nursing books will vary greatly in the particular methods shown for such proceedings as bandaging or dressing wounds. Much variation will depend on nurse training schools, senior nursing staff and consultants' likes and dislikes. It is important to remember that because methods vary, no one person may be right or wrong. Always ask yourself:

1 Does the procedure/method follow general guidelines, i.e. bandages should be applied joint to joint, aseptic technique maintained.
2 Does the procedure/method 'do the job' it is intended to, i.e. does the strapping support the ankle sprain? Does the sling support the arm correctly in the position required?
3 Is your patient as safe as possible, i.e. is the procedure/method you have been shown a safe method or does it put the patient's health or well being at risk?

If the answers are yes, then the various methods of applying a bandage or dressing a wound are not wrong, they are simply a variation on another's teaching.

It is hoped that with good management all staff within a department will be carrying out procedures using the same method but even this varies occasionally and certainly will vary from one department to another. Always have an open mind and be prepared to accept the various methods available to reach the same goal.

Remember we are all individuals

Throughout the day you will be presented with very different situations. You will find some days much busier than others. The number of patients seen per day is never an accurate means of determining the extent to which you will work. One patient may require many hours of your time, and you may only be able to deal with one or two patients at once. On the other hand you may spend only a few minutes with other patients and deal with several together. The important fact is to always remember to deal with all patients as individuals, who must be cared for as such. Each person will have different needs and problems. Many conditions, for example fractures or wounds, will be dealt with in a similar manner but the disability and length of incapacity will be totally different. Unless we recognise the individual we will not be able to deal with the many problems that can arise.

The whole nursing care of patients in Accident & Emergency must reflect the total person with individual needs and problems. This does not only relate to the patient's physical condition or psychological state. It includes the patient's home environment, relatives and ability to cope with his or her condition.

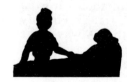

Many departments have 'regular' customers who call in for companionship, describing some fictitious disorder in order to be permitted to spend time in the Waiting Room chatting to other patients. Many people expect the Accident & Emergency department to solve their marital or housing arrangements – you will be surprised how many people, after an argument with their spouse, suddenly develop a condition that warrants hospital care; once given a clean bill of health they will tell you the real reason for coming.

The elderly lady who is admitted to hospital

may be more concerned about her cat than herself. Her cat is a very important problem to her which must be dealt with. You may meet patients and relatives who are uncooperative and unwilling to listen to reason; these people must be dealt with in a courteous manner despite their attitude.

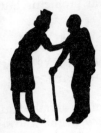

Many patients will respond to a learner's approach and often patients will open themselves to the junior nurse more readily than to the Sister or doctor. If patients do confide in you your response will obviously depend on the situation, but often you can reassure them that you can help, even if this help is putting them in touch with the correct people. The lonely person with the fictitious disorder may well benefit from help from many of the voluntary organisations in the community. The marital or housing problem may be dealt with through the appropriate authorised bodies or the hospital Social Work Department.

Patients with injuries such as a fracture will have to cope suddenly with new needs and problems. The forty year old man may now be unable to work, and this may cause financial embarrassment. He may live alone and have difficulty with his home and cleaning arrangements. Perhaps he has an elderly parent who depends on him to physically help with his daily needs. The seventy year old woman may have extremely arthritic legs and rely on her arms for holding onto walls and fences when walking. Perhaps she uses a walking aid. This lady may be totally unable to manage in her own home with one arm in plaster.

These illustrate some of the many unique problems and needs you will see in the Accident & Emergency department. We cannot treat any patient just for their apparent condition but must consider the total person. Much help can be provided through the Accident & Emergency department in the form of Social

Services, home nursing, Meals on Wheels, home help and, if necessary, admission to a ward due to the inability to cope because of the injury. This help can only be arranged if we recognise all the problems correctly. This means that during assessment of every person you should consider all aspects so that you can identify not only their actual problems but also potential ones.

What does the Accident & Emergency Department offer you, the learner?

What the staff of the department should aim to achieve is to provide you with the knowledge and skills to cope with a variety of injuries and illness, some minor, some major. You will see for the first time the many ways patients present with their acute medical or surgical conditions. You will understand the need for good communication between the departmental staff and Social Workers, District Nurse, Liaison Officers, Pre-hospital Services (Ambulance, Police and Fire), and the liaison that must exist between the department and the wards, X-ray, Theatre and many other departments and personnel within the hospital. Most importantly you will learn how to deal with many patients rapidly, how to develop professional relationships with patients for short periods of time and to gain their confidence and trust. The Accident & Emergency department is not isolated; in fact it is the centre of patient care from the time the patient enters through the doors until their discharge or admission to the ward.

The inter-relationships with other areas and the A & E department

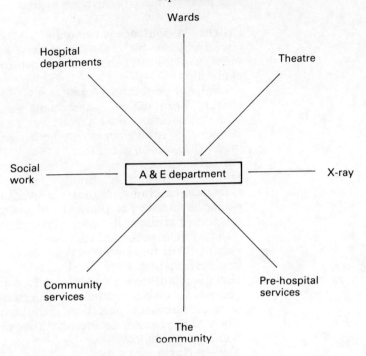

Communication

This is the key word in any Accident & Emergency department. Communication is so important because it is unlikely that one person will deal with the patient from arrival to admission or discharge. It would be ideal if one nurse could follow a patient through all the stages of care – assessment, intervention, evaluation and discharge or admission – but in reality this is rarely possible. What often occurs is that the patient will be dealt with by several people and all must communicate with each other. Records should be kept up-to-date with all relevant information recorded.

Let us look at the number of communication links required for just one patient:

Patient – Ambulance personnel
History of present complaint, initial assessment, worries and fears. Reassurance and explanation.

Ambulance personnel – Nurse
History from patient, assessment made at scene. Condition during journey. Relative situation (who lives nearby, whether any are present). Home environment.

Patient – Nurse
Further history if required, more detailed assessment including clinical observation. Explanation for need to undress and gown. Description and disposal of property (explain that hospital does not accept liability). Needs of patient identified, intervention commenced. Explanation to patient at all stages of care. Encourage questioning. Answers to patient's questions. Check patient's understanding. Correct discharge procedure and giving of advice if the Doctor decides that they may go home.

Nurse – Nurse
Explanation of patient's physical and psychological problems and needs. Social situation. Presence or absence of relatives. Intervention required. Update at all stages of care. Often one nurse will not deal with the patient throughout; when handing over to other nurses, a complete report is required, including history obtained from ambulance personnel and intervention to date.

Nurse – Doctor
History from ambulance personnel, history to date, clinical observation. Nursing intervention carried out. Medical intervention prescribed, plan of treatment explained. Assist with medical intervention and question if unsure of needs.

Doctor – Patient
A more detailed medical examination, family history. Past medical history. Explanation of possible diagnosis, treatment, length of stay in hospital, referral system.

Doctor – Doctor
Referral and request consultation. Full history and medical findings. Possible diagnosis.

Doctor – Relatives
History if required, explanation of medical findings, diagnosis and line of treatment.

Nurse – Relatives
Back up of explanation given, further explanation as necessary. Reassurance. Inform about visiting times, requirements for patient's stay.

Doctor – Ward staff
Condition and diagnosis of patient. Intervention required on ward. General condition of patient at present.

Nurse – Ward staff
Full step by step care given in Accident & Emergency. Situation of relatives – whether

Communication is vital

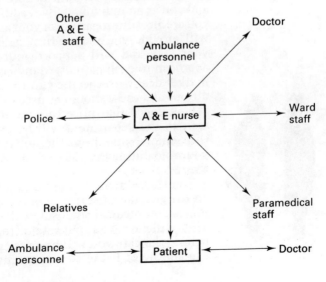

present, not contacted or gone home. Property
– what is with patient, what is in the safe, what
has been taken by relatives. Complete evaluation of patient with ward staff.

It can be seen from the diagram that the
Accident & Emergency nurse is central to all
communication within the department. If
communication broke down at this level,
patient care would be at risk. It is essential that
communication at all stages of patient care is
maintained. Remember also that all history,
problems identified through assessment and
step by step intervention must be recorded on
the patient's record charts.

All communication must be a two-way process. Nurses must listen, ask questions and
explain. It is essential that the patient understands all explanations given and the nurse
should reinforce these as necessary.

Preparation for Allocation

This will depend on your School of Nursing
and you as an individual. By reading this book
you are already preparing for your allocation, it
will provide you with a firm framework for
your stay and will support your individual
approach to each patient. Many books on the
market deal with specific clinical care of conditions and these should be used as necessary.

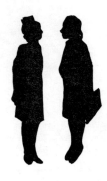

It is hoped that prior to your allocation, a
visit to the department will be arranged and
the Senior Nurse from the unit will explain
your role during the time you are allocated to
them.

You should refresh your current knowledge
on the general nursing care of patients suffering acute medical and surgical conditions.
This will help you understand the rationale
behind the care you will observe and provide.
The following list of conditions may help; all

those given are commonly seen in patients coming to the department and require immediate nursing intervention:

Head injury
Loss of consciousness
Diabetics (especially hypoglycaemia)
Cerebrovascular accidents
Multiple injury
Chest pain (cardiac and non-cardiac)
Overdose of drugs
Cardiac arrest
Fractures
Febrile convulsions and epilepsy
Gynaecological conditions
Psychiatric disorders

You can also use this list as a guide for further reading and questions while in the department.

Bandages and Strappings

Many books provide detailed instructions on how to apply the various types of bandages and strapping used in Accident & Emergency. Very few are used in the ward environment, so this is a new skill which must be acquired. Although these books are useful, it should be remembered that there is often more than one correct method for a particular application and each department will favour one method over another; it is important therefore that you are guided by the staff of the unit so that uniformity of application is achieved.

General rules are necessary to prevent complications developing when applying bandages and strapping. All bandages and strapping should be from joint to joint, e.g. base of the toes to just below the knee if supporting an ankle injury. This should also apply when dealing with lower leg injuries. A wound mid lower leg, especially in the elderly, will often be difficult to heal. This is frequently due to poor blood supply, especially with thin tissue-like skin flap injuries. Oedema often accompanies this. If the dressing is applied over the wound and the bandage only applied to this area, gross oedema occurs below and above the wound and healing is delayed.

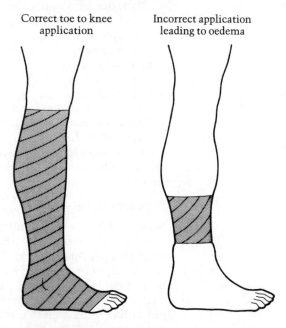

Correct toe to knee
application

Incorrect application
leading to oedema

The bandage or strapping should do the job it is intended for. It is no use, when the patient arrives at the bus stop having been discharged, to find the bandage intended to support the knee is round the ankle, having been incorrectly applied. This also does not do the image of nursing and the department any good. Conversely, the strapping applied for a sprained ankle should not be so tight as to cause circulatory problems to the foot.

Patients should always be advised that if a bandage or strapping becomes loose or tight, they should seek advice from the department or return for adjustment. Elasticated strapping around limbs can be hazardous and patients should be advised to watch fingers or toes for colour change, any feeling of numbness, tingling or swelling – any of these occurring should be reported.

If plaster of Paris has been applied, the patient should be instructed to watch for similar problems and return immediately they occur.

Your First Week

The first week of any allocation is always the worst. You feel lost and perhaps no more so than in the Accident & Emergency department. Gone are the familiar daily routines of the ward and that reassuring knowledge that although patients and their ailments are different, ward care of patients is somewhat similar. It is essential that learners are allocated to trained staff and allowed to settle into this new environment. Many departments have either a one–one allocation or have designated staff to look after new learners. Ideally the trained nurse and the learner should work the same duty rota for at least the first two weeks, so that continuity of teaching is maintained.

From day one you should be looking into every cupboard and drawer, especially areas where emergency equipment is kept. You should also begin to familiarise yourself with how various pieces of equipment work and are correctly cleaned.

During this week you should practise, under supervision, applying the various bandages, strappings and other unfamiliar dressings. Suturing is a very common procedure undertaken by medical or trained nursing staff. You must, therefore, become knowledgeable and capable of preparing equipment and assisting with this. Testing the visual acuity of patients with eye conditions is another simple skill you will need to acquire.

Care of patients' property is a vital part of nursing in the Accident & Emergency department. Many patients dealt with in a hurry can lose their property and many are not able, due to their condition, to care for their own property. Therefore we must be responsible. It is a very important part of total care of a patient to also care for their property; what may appear unimportant to us may not be so for the patient.

Most departments will have a procedure book filled with correct methods of coping with specific situations, particular conditions, application of bandages, emergency procedure for fire, cardiac arrest and much other useful information. You should, during this first

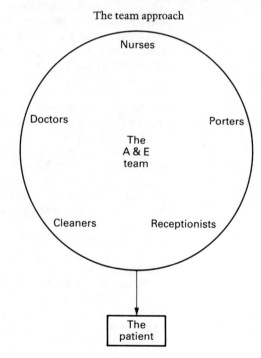

The team approach

week, begin to delve into this book and use it as reference.

In summary it is a very busy week, but enjoyable. You will soon begin to find your feet and become a part of the team, because this is what Accident & Emergency is about, a team approach – doctors, nurses, receptionists, porters, cleaners are all part of one team with one purpose – to offer an efficient and professional service to everyone who comes through our doors.

During your stay

As your weeks of allocation progress, you will learn how to correctly undress an injured patient and what position is best for certain conditions or injuries. You should study the various complaints that patients present with and become familiar with the kinds of nursing care which may be required, including observation and assessment and the overall care of the patient from arrival in the department to admission or discharge.

Whenever possible you should follow a patient's care from start to finish. This will include:

Assessment of patient's condition
Identifying actual and potential problems
Understanding and dealing with the care of the patient (intervention)
Evaluating the patient's progress and your own actions.

You will be responsible for the following:

Correct undressing of patient
Care of property
Clinical observation
Care of relatives
Organisation of specific observation by other paramedical staff
Obtaining records as necessary

Assisting the doctor and observing the proceedings

Carrying out specific nursing and prescribed medical care

Accompanying patient to the ward or help with discharge

Cleaning and replacing equipment used.

Your nursing skills will develop as the weeks progress and usually after the first two to three weeks you should have acquired a very broad concept of Accident & Emergency work.

You are now in a position to start looking in greater detail at individual patients, the problems they present with, the correct assessment and care of these people and their expected outcome (goal). Many situations in which you will become involved are unique to Accident & Emergency departments, while many are inter-related with the law and you as a learner should take interest in all these situations. However, when it comes to the law or patient advice, it is always wise to refer to a trained Accident & Emergency nurse. As a learner you cannot take on this responsibility.

Police in Accident & Emergency

Patients involved in a road traffic accident will always be seen at some stage by a police officer. This is not necessarily to lay blame; the police are also concerned to help the person, who may be hundreds of miles from home and now without a car. Having said this, the police also have an obligation in law to obtain facts of an accident and, if alcohol is involved, to discover if this is in excess. Although the patient's care is of prime importance, nursing staff should always try to help police officers in their duty. Where a conflict may develop between what is good for the patient over what is required by the police, the patient's care always takes precedence. Good liaison between the two services, the hospital and the police, usually provides help for both patient and community.

When patients die of their injuries, or are brought in dead, the police are again involved. Any sudden death or death within 24 hours of admission to hospital is investigated by the Local Coroner. A Coroner's Officer is appointed to act on behalf of and with the Coroner. This person is a police officer and will always be involved in this situation. Relatives should be reassured and explanation given that this will occur, and that it does not suggest that any criminal act has taken place. Many relatives, if not prepared by nursing staff, may feel guilt at the sudden death. This only increases their dreadful situation and should be avoided by proper explanation from the staff.

Nurses should not wash bodies and 'lay out' the person as in the ward situation, as this could remove vital evidence. An enthusiastic nurse with soap and water may remove the only evidence the police and pathologist have of determining the cause of death.

Police may also come to the department to enquire after a patient's condition or attendance. Every department should have specific procedures on this and as a learner you should refer these enquiries to trained nursing staff.

It is an unfortunate fact of life that terrorism and riots are becoming a much more common part of our day to day lives. The police involvement in such situations is immense. Co-operation with police at these times not only helps the victims but also the community as a whole. To identify the exact nature of a car bomb the police often need details of which pieces of shrapnel come from which area of the patient's body. Continuity of evidence can be achieved if nurses, during the undressing process, bag clothes separately and where possible identify the location from whence certain items of foreign matter have been removed. Care should be taken not to remove evidence. Even soiled dressings applied at the scene could be useful, so save and bag everything. Always clearly label all items with the patient's name. Clothes, if cut for removal, should, where possible, not be cut through the holes or tears inflicted by an instrument, e.g. a knife or foreign body. This again aids the investigation.

Inner City Problems

Although rape, drug abuse and civil disruption can occur in any area of the country or world, it is often much more common in inner city areas. Drug abuse is a major problem and if you are working in an inner city hospital it is not uncommon to meet on a daily basis the victims of it. Most hospitals who have a large drug addicted population will already be organised in the care of these patients. They may have designated areas where addicts can 'sleep off' the effect of their evening's activity.

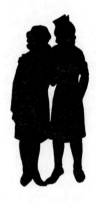

Rape is a very horrific occurrence for a woman and a large amount of understanding and sympathy is required should a victim present to the department. She will usually wish to inform the police, though this is not always the case. Encouragement to report such an incident must be handled carefully as fear of accusation is often one reason for failure to report to the police. Examination will be conducted by the police surgeon or a gynaecologist. The presence of female nurses is a great help to the patient during this very distressing situation.

Civil unrest either on a small or large scale is seen in areas of deprivation, usually in inner city areas. Nursing staff are becoming more aware of the need to split groups within the department in order to prevent the street fight continuing there.

Infection

Nurses in Accident & Emergency are always at risk from infection. Correct hygiene by the nurse and use of protective clothing and gloves when required will greatly reduce this risk. Always remember that in this department you do not know your patient's history. For example, you have no idea if the blood contains Hepatitis B virus. Pyrexia of unknown origin can be due to a fairly harmless flu virus or lassa fever; you do not know and it is therefore wise to take certain precautions:

1   Always be careful of blood or other body fluids. Wear gloves when appropriate and always wash your hands carefully.
2   Patients with pyrexia of unknown origin should be barrier nursed until proven safe.
3   If you injure yourself with a sharp implement, such as a dirty needle or blade, report immediately to a doctor and follow your hospital policy for such occurrences.
4   Use a recommended solution to wash blood or other body fluids from trolleys or work surfaces. Sodium hypochlorite is the solution of choice.

Non-Accidental Injury

Non-accidental injury to children is seen, often for the first time, in the Accident & Emergency department. Many such children are identified by the vigilance of the department's staff. Many parents will present with very convincing stories regarding the injury of their child. The staff must listen carefully and

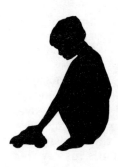

consider if this injury corresponds totally with the story. Many parents may not have deliberately injured their child, but through neglect or inexperience caused injury. It is important that staff are watchful but not paranoid; suspicion of every parent would be a dreadful situation. If you as a learner think that a child's injuries are suspicious, you should refer the situation immediately to a trained nurse who will proceed according to the policy for child abuse within your department. Many tell-tale signs can make one wary – injuries that do not relate to the history, parents who may appear in conflict, the child who appears distant from one or other parent, the sometimes absurd stories parents will give as the cause of the injury, bruises on other areas of the body, a torn mouth frenulum. These are just a few of the signs you should be watching for during the assessment of the child.

The Violent and Potentially Violent Patient

Some patients in the Accident & Emergency department may become violent. This violence is often of a verbal nature, but can become physical. While much is attributed to alcohol, it can also be due to psychiatric disorders, physical conditions and plain aggression on the patient's part.

Stress of waiting times, worry about relatives who are injured and the approach of the staff can all affect the situation. The attitude of the staff will often change a potentially violent situation, for better or worse. Many people come in worried and concerned about their own condition or that of relatives. Correct assessment and explanation *on arrival* is essential. Time must be given to each person; one major nursing skill to be developed here is the ability to interact with numerous patients at once yet allow each patient the benefit of being an individual. This is not easy. On many days you will feel pressured by the number of patients; at this point if one person appears uncooperative, demanding or aggressive, it is all too easy to show hostility. It then becomes easy for violence, verbal or physical, to occur. Your attitude must be one of calm, interest and explanation; this may not always work but more times than not it will and you can pat yourself on the back for suppressing a developing situation.

Now you are ready

Well, perhaps you are ready at least for the other chapters of this book. Remember the majority of people have never attended a hospital before, they are injured or have injured or sick relatives. They, like you, are nervous; they, like you, are looking for a reassuring smile, a helping hand, an explanation as to what is happening. They also, in the majority of cases, are going home; therefore they need correct instructions as to how to continue treating their problem. The burn to the foot will heal more rapidly if it is elevated at home. The axilla will not become sore and present an odour if gently washed and powdered despite not removing the sling. Wounds will heal with sutures if the patient is instructed not to get them wet or, for a finger wound, not to continuously wear a plastic finger cover so the perspiration soaks the skin. The patient will return, perhaps the next day but this relies on you remembering to arrange an appointment before they leave. They, of course, may return before then if they have not been told all these things or not had sufficient explanation that the crepe bandage does not cure a sprained ankle in 24 hours, or if they must see their doctor for further advice or treatment. Remember, you need help and guidance, as does the patient, because we are all individuals.

2 Triage and the Nursing Process

It is very difficult to separate the nursing process from triage as both are so closely linked. Assessment is the key factor in both and it is essential that this is performed by an experienced Accident & Emergency nurse.

Nursing Process

The basic principles of this remain the same, whether undertaken in the ward environment or the Accident & Emergency department. It is a logical systematic approach to nursing involving individual nurse/patient interaction. It is a knowledgeable, purposeful series of thoughts and actions encompassing:

Assessment
Identifying actual and potential problems
Goal setting and nurse intervention
Evaluation

Various adaptations of this approach exist and each department may well differ in the particular model used. Many may not use a specific model of care but use the four headings above and record the care under these headings.

This book is based on the use of the four major headings produced in separate chapters to allow the nurse to use each chapter for reference, if wished.

Assessment

This step in the process of care involves the collection of information gathered:

1 in the nursing history, and
2 by signs and symptoms presented.

A clear history is essential, for example:

'Was the patient unconscious before he fell down the stairs?'

'Did he shout as he fell and then become unconscious at the bottom after striking his head?'

'Does the patient live alone and will she find difficulty going home?'

'Could the patient walk before the accident or is this a new problem?'

'Was the tablet bottle full or were there only two tablets left?'

Signs and symptoms, with the history, help the nurse to make a full assessment of the patient's problems. Signs are what the nurse can see, symptoms are what the patient tells the nurse. Pain, inability to move, visual disturbance and a feeling of nausea are all symptoms. Pale skin, deformity and swelling are all signs. For example, a *history* of sudden collapse to the ground and *signs* of pale or cyanosed skin and no chest movement indicate an *assessment* that respiratory arrest is present.

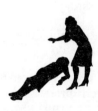

Identifying Actual and Potential Problems

This part of the process involves identifying a patient's actual or potential need which requires nursing action. This stage cannot be reached without an accurate assessment. Analysis of the data collected at the assessment stage will enable the nurse to clearly identify all problems. It must be emphasised that unless correct assessment has taken place, this stage will not be achieved and the following stages of care will also be adversely affected.

Goal Setting and Nurse Intervention

The nurse must state a specific result she wishes to reach due to nursing action. In turn, the nurse intervention must be such that the goals (result) required will be achieved. Within the Accident & Emergency department the goals and intervention will be based on:

1 The assessment and problems identified
2 The accident and emergency knowledge of the nurse
3 The doctor's plan of action

Evaluation

This final step in the process of care is essential. It is the periodical review of the patient's response to the nursing actions. By evaluation of the response, new problems, goals and intervention are identified. The nurse can determine if the goals have been achieved; if they have not, she will be able to alter the plan to meet the patient's new or original needs.

When evaluating, the nurse must always bear in mind:

Are the goals logical; are they achievable?
Do the nursing approaches indicate: What is to be done? When it is to be done? Who is to do it?

Having looked briefly at the nursing process and its major components, we must now discuss how this can be implemented within the department. The hospital where you work may have formal nursing process forms; however, it must be remembered that the forms and charts are a means of recording your care. They do not of themselves change your individual approach to patients and their problems.

Ideally the department will have some means of recording your assessment, problems, action and evaluation. This may be the same form as used on the ward, or it may be specifically designed for the department. The

One approach to documenting the care of a patient in the A & E department

			ORSETT ACCIDENT AND EMERGENCY RECORD FORM			

NAME: **AGE:**   Date and time of admission to A&E

NEXT OF KIN: NAME   **RELATIVES INFORMED:**   Yes/No

Tel. No.:

Address of N of K:

ADMISSION observation and history of today's problem:

P	B/P	T	R	D/S	Urine	
					X-rays	
					ECG	
					Bloods	

Allergies:

ASSESSMENT: – How does patient look/feel:

A/E Nurses Signature:

PROBLEMS – tick:

Chest pain	Diabetic	Fitting	OTHERS – please state:
Abdo pain	Vomiting	Head inj.	
Shortness of breath	Headaches	Limb inj.	
Bleeding PV	History of un/consc.	Back pain	
	Unconscious		

ACTION	EVALUATION	SIG.
Bed rest – position		

ACTION	EVALUATION	SIG.

	ADMISSION FORM	
CLOTHING	IN GREY BAG	
	GIVEN TO RELATIVE/FRIEND	
DENTURES	NONE	
	IN PATIENT'S MOUTH	
	IN DENTURE POT	
	GIVEN TO RELATIVE/FRIEND	
SPECTACLES	NONE	
	PATIENT WEARING	
	IN BAG	
	GIVEN TO RELATIVE/FRIEND	
VALUABLES	NONE	
	HANDED IN FOR SAFE KEEPING	
	GIVEN TO RELATIVE/FRIEND	
	WITH PATIENT	

OTHER SPECIFY:

Signed . . . .

Signed . . . .
(Ward Nurse)

forms must be easy to use in a fast moving area and should not be so complex as to require long periods of nursing time to fill them in. A standard care plan is used in some Accident & Emergency departments to increase speed. If not handled correctly, however, it can become a ritual plan implemented for every patient. This has the serious disadvantage of losing the individual approach to the patient's problem.

Forms should have sufficient space to record the nurse's assessment; ideally a standard Accident & Emergency record has combined nursing and medical care. Where separate forms are used, these can also include a property check as many situations in the department can lead to claims of lost property.

It is essential, whatever type of form or record sheet is in use, that nurses record all assessment, intervention and evaluation. One nurse may not follow a patient through all areas of care, so good record keeping is essential for efficient individual care.

Triage

Triage indicates the care, sets the pace and controls the flow of patients within the department. The word *triage* originates from the French meaning to pick, sort, select. It has been used by military personnel for many years, the procedure being first described in the military history of World War I as a 'Triage or Sorting Station'. Use of triage in the Accident & Emergency department has been slowly adopted within the UK. In the USA triage in Emergency departments began around 1963; since then the person undertaking triage has varied from physician to nurse, from volunteer to paramedic. It is now generally accepted that triage in the Accident & Emergency departments requires the skills of an experienced nurse familiar with the resources and constraints within the department. In the UK many departments still allow Reception Staff to triage patients; this triage falls into two categories:

Category 1: Those who are bleeding or collapsing at the Reception Desk
Category 2: All others

This use of Reception Staff is quite unacceptable as the majority of patients fall into Category 2 and consequently sit sometimes for hours in the waiting room having seen neither a nurse nor a doctor. All patients should be seen on arrival by a nurse. This allows assessment to be undertaken and priorities of care to be established. The methods used to establish a functional triage service will depend on the department's geography, nursing establishment and most importantly the commitment of staff to the system.

In the department where you are about to work you may find a nurse allocated to a triage desk in the waiting room. Other departments use assessment rooms or the patient comes to an assessment/triage area. The method used is of little consequence; what is important is that the goals of triage are achieved:

1   Early patient assessment
2   Determination of urgency of need for care
3   Control of patient flow
4   Assignment to correct area of care
5   Initiation of diagnostic measures

Assessment

This has been discussed earlier and the chapter relating to assessment gives guidelines as to correct patient assessment.

Determination of Urgency of Need

Although Platt in 1962 removed the word 'Casualty' to be replaced with 'Accident &

Emergency', a vast number of patients attending the department do not require immediate care. Many may require urgent or semi-urgent care and some can be delayed until time and staff are available to see them.

The type of urgency rating system will differ in each Department.

System I
A two category system – Urgent and Non-urgent.

The trained nurse assessing patients may use this chart as one guide but must make a priority rating on the patient's presenting condition

Priority 1 (red)
Any patient who has potential life threatening conditions affecting airway, breathing or circulation or whose condition will deteriorate very rapidly if not seen and treated. This will include any patient who has an injury or condition where hypovolaemia or cardiogenic shock is evident or due to the injuries/condition is likely to occur, i.e.:
Multiple injury
Severe head injury
Laceration with exaggerated bleeding
Large % burns or scalds, i.e. above 10–15%
Patients in convulsion
Unconscious patients
Overdose
Chest pains where cardiac condition is likely

Priority 2 (yellow)
Patients who need to be seen urgently but a short wait will not result in threat to life.
Probable fractures (pain, deformity)
Probable dislocations
Embedded foreign bodies, i.e. fish hooks
Epistaxis which is still bleeding
Varicose veins which are bleeding
Burns and scalds
Unwell children Post febrile convulsion
Road traffic accident (RTAs) multiple abrasions, bruises, etc.
Head injury: drowsy, history of loss of consciousness
Acute neck pain and injury
Eye injuries or foreign bodies
Psychological or social 'trouble' who need to get out of department

Priority 3 (green)
Patients who can wait for any length of time (within reason) without their condition being affected.
Second opinion from G.P. or patient.
Follow up not at correct time.
Long standing complaints, i.e. ankle injury, back ache, etc. more than 24 hours old.
Old wounds, boils, etc.
Minor injuries, i.e. tiny abrasions, just for tetanus, etc.
General check-ups, i.e. have not been well for months.
'Thought I would call because I work weekdays.'
Children who look fine but have been 'unwell' for weeks.
Ankle injuries, limb injuries with no obvious major injury.

System II
A three category system – Immediate, Urgent, Delayed.

System III
A five category system – Immediate, Urgent, Semi-urgent, Delayed, No need for care.

System II (three categories) is the most widely used system but much will depend on the number of patients using the department and the type of variety of patients seen. Colour coding is often used – Red for Immediate, Yellow for Urgent, Green for Delayed.

The system should be flexible to allow movement of patients from one category to another, depending on the continuous evaluation that should take place. Use of protocols and descriptive clinical states allow the nurse to place the patient in the correct category.

Examples of how patients should be correctly triaged:
Laceration:

Assessment	Area of injury
	Mechanism of injury
	Amount of bleeding, type of bleeding
	Extent of wound contamination
Intervention	Depends on assessment but will include covering wound with sterile dressing
Urgency rating	If heavy or arterial bleeding (Priority 1)
	If able to control with dressing but is deep and contaminated (Priority 2)
	If minor abrasion with superficial damage only (Priority 3)

Chest pain:

Assessment	Type of pain
	Area of pain
	If associated with movement
	If persistent or intermediate
	Any history of injury
	Signs of cardiogenic shock
Intervention	Depends on assessment
Urgency rating	If suggestive of cardiac origin (Priority 1)
	If history of injury and no shortness of breath (Priority 2)
	If associated with movement and old injury (Priority 3)

Explanation to Patients

Explanation of the triage system to patients on arrival is essential. People will usually accept a reasonable explanation of why they have to wait if delegated to Priority 3. Invitation should always be given to return to the triage area should the patient feel the need for re-assessment, i.e. blood is coming through the bandage, child becoming drowsy. When re-assessed, the priority rating may remain the same or may be changed. A child having been hit on the head may well have been placed in Priority 2 – Urgent. A sudden loss of consciousness while waiting to be seen would move the child to Priority 1 – Immediate.

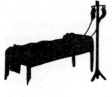

Urgency rating will also change depending on the department's activity; patients placed in the Immediate category may well be moved to Urgent if a more serious life threatening condition arose in another patient. This is seen clearly in the major incident situation where patients who on a normal daily basis would be considered Immediate or Urgent may well be placed in a much lower category.

Another method of categorising patients is by the nature of their medical condition, e.g. cardiac related chest pain would need the attention of the physician. Chest pain related to trauma would need surgical intervention. In some departments nurses undertaking triage are allowed to perform such categorisation, as well as using the urgency rating.

Patient/Nurse	Gynaecology	Priority 1 Priority 2 Priority 3
	Paediatrics	Priority 1 Priority 2 Priority 3
	Medical	Priority 1 Priority 2 Priority 3
	Psychiatric	Priority 1 Priority 2 Priority 3

Control of Patient Flow

This is part of the managerial structure of the department. The triage nurse must maintain control over trolley areas and know the present position and occupancy of all areas within the department.

Assignment to Correct Area of Care

Once priority rating has been established, the triage nurse must decide the most appropriate area of care. Many patients will be allocated to the Waiting Area as their priority rating will be delayed or semi-urgent. Patients with a priority rating of 1 (immediate care) must be assigned to the correct area for the care of their condition, i.e. resuscitation area for cardiac arrest.

Initiation of Diagnostic Measures

Although in the USA this would refer to blood tests and other extensive investigations, in the UK it is restricted to nursing observation where nurse intervention may well be required. Temperature, pulse, respiration and blood pressure, electrocardiograph and blood sugar estimation plus urine testing are the types of diagnostic measurements undertaken at the triage point.

The Nurse Learner at Triage

The nurse learner's role at the triage desk or office should be one of observation and assistance. It is at this area that you will gain your major insight into patient assessment. Assessment at the point of triage will be brief; it can be divided into subjective and objective. Subjective assessment is how the patient sees the problem, what the patient tells you and what history is obtained. Objective assessment is what you as the nurse see, hear and feel when examining the patient and will include diagnostic measurements.

The degree to which the assessment is performed will be determined by the number of patients coming through the area at any one time.

At first it will appear an easy nursing skill to talk and obtain a history from a patient. It will appear easy to initiate priority rating and allocate specific areas of care. As you progress during your stay and realise the different presentations of many patients, you will begin to understand how complex the triage nurse's job is.

What to observe
Listen to the history from the patient.
Listen to the questions the nurse asks.
Observe the head to toe check.
Record and assimilate the results of diagnostic measurements.
Become familiar with triage records.

Observe priority rating and question the triage nurse on these ratings.

Observe and question the first aid care given at triage.

Observe the management aspect of the triage nurse in keeping the patient flow smooth.

Assistance at Triage

This will depend to what extent nurse learners act in the nursing care of patients in your Accident & Emergency department. When busy you should not be tempted to try and carry out triage alone; instead the assessment should be carried out by the trained nurse. You may undertake diagnostic measurements but these should be checked if found to be abnormal or inconsistent with the assessment. First aid care can often by implemented by you once the wound or injury has been seen by the triage nurse.

As you progress in experience the taking of history and assessment can be done with the triage nurse observing your skills. This method allows you to undertake triage in a safe environment knowing that any patient information missed by you will be noted by the trained nurse.

Combining Triage and the Nursing Process

Combining both triage and the nursing process, nurses within the Accident & Emergency department can provide the most effective service to the patient. A workable system requires first and foremost patient assessment on arrival. All patients when assessed can then be placed into priority rating.

The nurse who is allocated the patient from

the triage point then commences the nursing process. A more indepth assessment is performed and goals and intervention initiated. The nurse allocated to the patient area will constantly evaluate the patient's progress and re-assess goals and intervention as necessary. The triage nurse must be kept up-to-date with progress of each patient. Nursing records should be completed and reflect the care given during the patient's stay.

Example of Triage and Nursing Process Records

Triage:
1 Subjective assessment
Severe pain in chest, central and tight in nature; radiates to left arm.
2 Objective assessment
Pale, cold, clammy skin

Urgency rating 1 (Immediate)

Area of care: major Medical (Resusc.)

Nursing process:
Assessment Patient pale, cold and clammy skin. Pulse 110, weak but regular rhythm; BP 90/50; respiration 25, shallow but regular. Still complaining of severe tightness in chest and down left arm.

Problem Acute chest pain with associated cardiogenic shock.

Goal
1 To improve patient's cardiovascular state
2 Reduce chest pain

Intervention Obtain medical attention immediately. Nursed on chest bed, normally in semicircumbent position (45°) (allows 30% less cardiac work). Oxygen administered at 60% concentration (reduces incidence of arrhythmias). Monitor cardiac rhythm and record pulse, respiration and blood pressure every 15 minutes. Reassure patient and keep area quiet.

Evaluation Improved, pain much less since administration of analgesic. Pulse 90; BP 110/60; respiration 20. Skin dry and colour now slightly pink, some pallor around eyes remains. Continue oxygen and semicircumbent position. Has passed urine and no abnormalities detected.

3 Mrs Brown, an Individual Patient

One purpose of this book is to make you aware of all your patients, not as conditions in a cubicle, but as individual humans with individual problems, fears and worries.

This chapter takes you through one patient's care while in the Accident & Emergency department. Although perhaps tomorrow you will meet another person with similar injuries, because of everyone's individuality the other person may require totally different care and intervention.

Assessment

Mrs Brown arrived by ambulance early on Wednesday afternoon. While shopping she had fallen and injured her leg. The history from the ambulance staff indicated that Mrs Brown was complaining of a very painful hip and was unable to stand. From this it was decided to nurse Mrs Brown on a care trolley so movement would be restricted and in case an X-ray should be required.

As Mrs Brown was wheeled into the cubicle the nurse greeted her with a smile, indicating that she cared and would make her as comfortable as possible. Once Mrs Brown had been gently lifted onto the trolley by the ambulance staff, the nurse took a further history and made a complete head to toe examination. Pulse and blood pressure readings were recorded to obtain a base level and also to assess the general cardiovascular state. These were within acceptable levels. Had the pulse been rapid and the blood pressure low, internal bleeding would have been suspected and immediate action taken.

When the nurse was confident that no other injury was present, she undressed Mrs Brown with help and helped her into a hospital gown. Mrs Brown was advised to take nothing by mouth until a doctor had completed the examination (should a fracture be present, surgical intervention may be required).

Mrs Brown appeared more concerned over her son than herself. Brian Brown suffers from Down's syndrome. Brian will be leaving school at 3.30 pm and is always met by his mother. Foreseeing great difficulties if she were not there, Mrs Brown was very anxious to leave the hospital despite the pain in her hip. Assessment had thus not only revealed Mrs Brown's physical problems but also the concern and anxiety over her son in time to make other arrangements.

| GOALS | 1 Reduction of pain in hip |
| | 2 Collection of son from school |

NURSING CARE

Intervention

Having undressed Mrs Brown carefully, the nurse supported her injured leg by pillows at either side. Mrs Brown felt more comfortable lying flat with one pillow for her head; this position was therefore maintained. The support and position reduced tension on the hip muscles thus greatly decreasing pain.

Mrs Brown gave a neighbour's telephone number to the nurse who was checking property. Unfortunately the plan to ask the neighbour to collect Brian failed when no answer was received. The school was con-

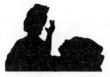

tacted directly and the problem explained. The teacher assured the nurse that she would look after Brian until a Social Worker from the hospital could collect him. The nurse had previously arranged with the Social Services in the hospital to collect Brian and bring him to the hospital. Each step in these arrangements was conveyed to Mrs Brown to allay her concern.

Medical examination was undertaken and an X-ray of the hip ordered. Mrs Brown was wheeled to the X-ray department but not removed from the trolley. After her return the medical staff reviewed both Mrs Brown and her X-ray result. Fortunately no fracture was present. Generalised bruising to the hip was diagnosed and a plan of action made to admit Mrs Brown for bed rest and then further physiotherapy. This course of treatment was explained to Mrs Brown, but rejected by her because of her concern for Brian's care.

Brian arrived in the department with the Social Worker; he was very distressed and immediately ran to his mother's side. Although he was only twelve years old, Brian was a well built, tall boy who was obviously very active. Mrs Brown indicated that Brian could be very boisterous and would not settle even if the neighbours agreed to look after him for a few days. Suggestion of care in a community home was greeted with horror despite the Social Worker's reassurance. Mrs Brown was adamant; home she would go. She would try to rest as much as possible.

At this point the medical staff can take one of two options, either formally discharge Mrs Brown and continue follow-up care as an outpatient, or consider this course unwise and ask Mrs Brown to sign a self-discharge form. Follow-up care as an outpatient would still be provided. Irrespective of the medical decision the nurse's role in this situation is to ensure that all assistance in the community is arranged.

The Social Worker was still present, and pointed out that through her Mrs Brown could have the support of the home help service and Meals on Wheels. The District Nurse Liaison Officer was called to the department and arrangements made for a nurse to call daily and a 'twilight nurse' to stop by in the evening to ensure that all was well. A commode and other aids such as a walking frame and bed cradle were organised through the Social Services.

Mrs Brown said that her neighbour would help out and some of the services may be cancelled as and when possible. Oral analgesia was prescribed by the doctor to take home and an outpatient's appointment booked. An ambulance came to transport her home. Further attempts to contact the neighbour were successful and she volunteered to help when Mrs Brown returned home.

Nursing intervention in this situation had involved not only the physical care of Mrs Brown but also meeting her psychological needs. Brian had been collected from school and reunited with his mother.

NURSING CARE

Evaluation

Having rested on a trolley with the leg supported the acute pain Mrs Brown was suffering on arrival had diminished to a dull ache. Thus one goal had been achieved. Brian had been collected from school and the reunion between mother and son not only helped Brian's psychological trauma but also reduced Mrs Brown's anxiety. The second goal had been achieved.

Organisation of the various social services and community nursing care had been satisfactorily arranged and transport home booked.

Mrs Brown, although realising the problem she faced with her painful hip and immobility, was much happier. Had the neck of the femur been fractured, the situation would have been totally different. Brian would have required care, Mrs Brown's anxiety would not have been allayed and nursing intervention would have had to be totally different.

4 Assessing Patients

Patients will arrive at the Accident &
Emergency department in a number of different ways. They may have made their own way
using bus, taxi, car or walking, or they may
have come via the Ambulance Service. Most
patients will have made the decision to attend
the department on their own, though some
will have been sent by their GP or from their
place of work.

On arrival within the department, irrespective of mode of transport or apparent condition, **All** patients must be assessed by a
nurse. This very important nursing procedure
should never be left to reception staff,
although good co-operation should always exist between the triage nurse and receptionist.
While the initial assessment is made by a
trained nurse, you should observe the skills
required and continue this assessment when
dealing with the patient. Assessment begins
immediately you see the patient arriving. Depending on your method within the department, the patient may book in at reception and
then be seen by a nurse, or the nurse may see
all patients before registration takes place.

The Walking Patient

This, the largest group of patients, has often
been the most neglected with regard to patient
assessment; often they are left for hours after
seeing the receptionist before being seen by
a nurse or doctor. Now, fortunately, in most

departments the patient is seen on arrival by a trained nurse. The initial meeting of patient and nurse should attempt to establish a trust and understanding. The patient, having had proper assessment and first aid care, is then able to wait until full medical assessment and treatment can be provided. This initial assessment and explanation reduce the possible irritation of patients within the waiting room and the nursing staff can work with the knowledge that patients waiting are able to do so without a serious deterioration in their condition.

HISTORY

Mr Smith arrived in the department one Saturday morning. He had driven in his car and felt rather embarrassed when explaining his problem to the receptionist. Mr Smith was complaining of a sore throat; he had tried to see his GP but the surgery had just closed. He realised it was not an emergency but it was very painful and he was concerned. After booking in, Mr Smith went to the Nursing Assessment Area. Mr Smith explained to the nurse there that he had developed a sore throat that morning. He felt generally weak and exhausted. The nurse asked further questions to help establish the exact problem and commenced clinical observation of temperature and pulse.

Mr Smith told the nurse that the pain in his throat woke him up at 3 am. He fell back to sleep but on waking this morning he still had a sore throat. The history of waking suddenly, due to the pain, caused the nurse to probe further and discover what Mr Smith was describing as a sore throat was in fact pain in the throat and neck. The nurse also observed that during this brief but essential assessment the skin colour of Mr Smith was becoming pale and he now had developed pain in his shoulders. The nurse enquired as to possible chest pain; there was no specific complaint of this nature. However, pain radiating from the heart may present in areas other than the chest, e.g. in the shoulders only. Mr Smith was placed on a trolley and further nursing observations of blood pressure and an electro-cardiograph were performed. The doctor was summoned immediately as the nurse had a suspicion that Mr Smith might be suffering a myocardial infarction; she was correct.

Myocardial infarction is the death of a portion of myocardium (heart muscle). Often referred to as a heart attack.

What this case history illustrates is how essential it is for nurses to assess all patients thoroughly upon arrival and to obtain a clear and detailed history. It would have been extremely easy for the nurse or receptionist to allow Mr Smith to sit, possibly hours, in the waiting room with what some may consider a non-emergency (sore throat); had that occurred, and had correct nursing assessment not been carried out, the outcome might have been very different for Mr Smith – cardiac arrest in the waiting room is no joke.

Although this is a true case history, it is not a common occurrence. It does illustrate how patients may present with very serious conditions but on arrival their signs and symptoms are minimal. Most walking patients are far less complicated but deserve the same attention and skill as was given to Mr Smith.

Limb Injuries

Injuries that present very commonly in any Accident & Emergency department are those involving limbs. Fractures, sprains, lacerations and burns are by far the most frequent injuries to limbs. There are, however, many other types of injury, such as dislocation of joints, crush injuries (mainly to fingers, hands and feet) and also major damage to limbs involving combinations of injuries, such as severe lacerations with compound fractures and accompanying nerve and blood vessel damage.

Assessment of the patient with a limb injury involves:

1   History of the injury
2   Length of time since occurrence

Specific assessment should always utilise a comparison between the injured and un-injured limb and include:

1   *Pulse* Is there a pulse distal to the injury? Absence of the pulse could indicate arterial obstruction. Fractures near joints such as the elbow are particularly hazardous to blood vessels. If arterial flow is affected, immediate intervention to re-establish blood flow to the limb is necessary.

2   *Colour of skin* Pale or cyanosed skin may indicate poor blood flow due to partial or total obstruction of blood vessels.

3   *Skin temperature* Decrease in skin temperature distal to the injury can indicate poor blood flow to the limb.

4   *Sensation* Lack of sensation could indicate sensory nerve damage; the extent of sensation loss would determine the intervention required.

5   *Imperfection of movement* Many patients with limb injuries will have imperfection of movement. This can be due to many reasons:

Fear – mainly due to pain
Pain even at rest
Motor nerve damage
Muscle damage
Bone damage
Joint damage/dislocation
Swelling/deformity
Ischaemia

6   *Swelling* Is there any obvious swelling? Most injuries to limbs produce some swelling. This swelling is due to increased blood flow to the injured area and loss of fluid into the

tissues. Although increased blood flow will aid healing, the initial outpouring of fluid into the tissues causes pain and imperfection of movement and suppresses healing.

7 *Is there a deformity?* Gross swelling causes difficulty for learners trying to identify whether deformity may be present. Deformity is due to the fracture site or dislocation being out of alignment.

8 *Is there a wound?* Wounds can be related or unrelated to bone injury. If there is a relationship this fracture is termed 'compound'. The risk is infection to the bone (osteomyelitis).

When assessing limb injury care with handling is important. The patient should never be forced to move an injured limb. Medical staff may attempt specific movements of the patient's limbs but nurses should assess only what the patient can or cannot achieve.

HISTORY

Mrs James, a seventy year old lady, arrived very tearful. Her daughter was very distressed, and in fact appeared more distressed than her mother. Mrs James had been walking up her garden when she tripped on a flagstone. Trying to stop herself from falling, she twisted her wrist under her body and her full weight pressed down on the wrist. This caused great pain. Having got up she found her wrist swollen and abnormally shaped, and had difficulty moving her fingers and wrist. Her daughter, concerned that Mum had 'broken' her wrist, called a neighbour and he drove them both to the hospital.

NURSING CARE

Assessment

When seen by the nurse in the Assessment Area, Mrs James was offered a seat and her daughter reassured. The nurse assessed Mrs James by first obtaining a history. While this was being done the nurse looked closely at the wrist and observed the swelling, deformity and lack of movement. The colour and warmth of the hand and fingers were noted. The radial pulse of the damaged wrist was felt indicating that the arterial blood flow had not been impaired. Mrs James was asked about the amount of pain she was experiencing and the arm was supported in a broad arm sling. The nurse also enquired when was the last time any food or drink had been taken and advised Mrs James not to eat or drink until all investigations and treatment had been carried out. (If a general anaesthetic is used to reduce the fracture it is essential that the stomach be empty to decrease the risk of vomiting and thus of inhaling vomit into the lungs.)

Once the obvious injury had been assessed the nurse was then in a position to discover if any other injury was present. Had Mrs James grazed her knees or elbow under her sleeve? Often minor injuries can be missed when one particular injury is so evident and causing the most pain. The nurse should also at this stage anticipate any problems that may arise while waiting for treatment and take action in the Assessment Area, for example, rings must be removed from fingers to prevent constriction with swelling. A gentle enquiry as to Mrs James' ability to cope with one arm injured will assist advance planning to involve the Social Services when treatment has been completed and discharge is imminent.

The nurse, having assessed Mrs James, must now decide on the priority of care required; this will depend on the result of the assessment:

1   Is the radial pulse present? (the pulse distal to the injury)
2   Is Mrs James in severe pain?
3   Is there obvious swelling and/or deformity?

Severe pain or circulatory obstruction are two major factors which would cause the nurse to place Mrs James in an urgent priority. Her age is also something that must be borne in mind – elderly people will often react more acutely to injury than will the young.

Intervention

Having fully assessed Mrs James and arranged her priority care, it is important that the nurse explain to her that the doctor will come as soon as possible. If she is feeling able to sit in the waiting room she may do so; often, however, elderly people can be quite shaken by such a fall and feel more secure resting on a stretcher trolley. Analgesia will often be prescribed in the form of an intramuscular injection; this both provides quick pain relief and still allows oral intake to be restricted. If Mrs James required analgesia she would never be left in the waiting room but made comfortable on a trolley.

Incorrect First Aid

On occasions, despite suffering a fairly serious injury, patients will be brought into the department walking. Often first aid has been incorrectly applied by workmates or the family.

Stephen was replacing a large plate glass window in a shop of the local town. He lost his balance and the glass caused an extensive wound to his lower arm. Blood poured from it. Stephen's workmate ran to him and tried to stop the bleeding with the use of his belt as a tourniquet. He then rushed Stephen to hospital, blood still dripping from the wound.

Assessment

On arrival in the Accident department, immediate assessment was undertaken by the nursing staff. The wound was quickly checked for any foreign body. (Had a foreign body been present, e.g. a piece of glass, the nurse would place pressure on the wound around the foreign body with the use of a ring pad of gauze. Never put pressure directly on a foreign body in the wound.) As no foreign body was observed, a pressure dressing was applied, the tourniquet removed, and the arm elevated. (Elevation of the arm using a high sling allows

Incorrect first aid

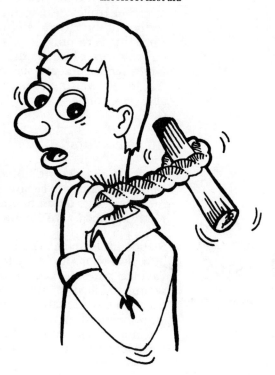

gravity to diminish the blood flow to the injured area. Pressure at the site of bleeding is the most effective method of stemming the flow of blood.)

The removal of the tourniquet allowed venous return to occur and lessened the congestion in the hand and arm. The length of time the tourniquet had been in place was noted on the record card. The radial artery had not been damaged and a strong radial pulse was present. Had the tourniquet been left on, arterial flow, in addition to venous circulation, would have been impaired. Nerve damage can also be caused by an incorrectly applied tourniquet. The prompt assessment by the nurse of the wound, correct first aid care, and removal of the tourniquet allowed Stephen to return home after suturing of his arm.

Head Injury

'My child has hit her head' – children are often brought to the Accident & Emergency department with this history and usually the parents are more concerned than the child. The assessment of patients with head injury must be detailed, and specific observations conducted. History taken from children is usually vague and an eye witness is often useful. Most patients with head injuries can be sent home after examination with instructions for relatives or friends to follow. These instructions are usually listed on a card. If the following symptoms occur they should be reported to a doctor or the patient should return to the department.

Severe headache	Irritability
Vomiting	Drowsiness
Double vision	Neck stiffness
Child continuously crying	Unconsciousness

Analgesia should also be avoided during the first twenty-four hours (this may mask symptoms).

HISTORY

Lisa arrived in a very quiet state, totally at variance to her normal happy, chatty self. Her mother gave a history of having seen Lisa fall from the swing in the garden. Lisa landed on the lawn and struck her head; she immediately cried and jumped up. Since then she had been very quiet and had also complained of some nausea but no vomiting.

NURSING CARE

Assessment

This history was important to the nurse assessing Lisa. Had the mother not been such a good historian, the nurse would have had to probe for these facts. It is extremely important to discover if a person who sustained a head injury was unconscious, even for a brief period after the event. This is because trauma sufficient to cause unconsciousness could also cause damage to blood vessels superficial to the brain (extradural). The vessels may bleed some hours after the injury causing increased intracranial pressure and possibly death if not detected at the early stages. Because Lisa had immediately cried and jumped up, no history of unconsciousness was apparent.

Having obtained the history, the nurse commenced neurological observations; these can be subdivided into what is termed the coma scale, the cardiovascular response, the pupils' response and limb movements.

Coma Scale

The Glasgow Coma Scale is the most widely used method of determining a patient's level of consciousness. It consists of three sections which are further subdivided:

1 Eyes open
   spontaneously
   to speech
   to pain
   none
2 Best verbal response
   orientated
   confused
   inappropriate words
   incomprehensible sounds
   none
3 Best motor response
   obey commands
   localise pain
   flexion to pain
   extension to pain
   none

Explanation such as semi-conscious means nothing as each nurse or doctor will interpret such an expression in a different manner.

The use of this method leaves no room for error and misinterpretation. The triage nurse was able to determine the exact level of consciousness which Lisa was presenting. She was sitting with her eyes open spontaneously, looking round the room. She knew her age, her name and where she lived. This indicated that she was orientated to time and place. It is important at this stage to confirm these details with Lisa's mother to ascertain whether the answers are correct. With an adult such questions should be avoided and questions such as date, environment, Prime Minister, current affairs, etc. should be asked; then there can be no confusion as to the correct answers.

Lisa was asked to lift her arms and point to the area on her head that hurt. She did this indicating that she heard and obeyed commands. From this assessment the nurse was happy that Lisa was conscious, orientated and able to understand and obey commands.

Cardiovascular response
This consists of counting and recording the pulse rate and recording the blood pressure.

(Decreased pulse rate and increased blood pressure could indicate increased intracranial pressure; however this is a late sign and this observation must be interpreted in the light of all other neurological findings.)

Pupils' response
Pupils should be equal in size and react when a light is shone into the eye. Reaction should be checked for both direct and consensual reflex. (The light shone into one eye will cause that pupil to react. The opposite pupil will also constrict due to nerve transfer. If sensory or motor nerve damage has occurred, one or other reflex may be absent.) Dilation of the pupil can occur on the side of injury if pressure within the skull is present.

While looking at the eyes, squint (strabismus) should be noted and recorded. It is also important if abnormal findings are present to determine if this is normal for the patient. Some people do have one pupil larger than the other. They may also have suffered a squint for years.

Limb movements
These are observed and recorded for arms and legs, left and right. The limb movements are sub-divided like the Coma Scale:
1 Arms (left and right)
   Normal power
   Mild weakness
   Severe weakness
   Spastic flexion
   Extension
   No response
2 Legs (left and right)
   Normal power
   Mild weakness
   Severe weakness
   Extension
   No response

Having completed the assessment the nurse will have a clear picture as to Lisa's neurological state and be able to make a decision on her priority.

NAME				DATE
RECORD No.				TIME

C O M A S C A L E	Eyes open	Spontaneously		Eyes closed by swelling = C
		To speech		
		To pain		
		None		
	Best verbal response	Orientated		Endotracheal tube or tracheostomy = T
		Confused		
		Inappropriate Words		
		Incomprehensible		
		None Sounds		
	Best motor response	Obey commands		Usually record the best arm response
		Localise pain		
		Flexion to pain		
		Extension to pain		
		None		

Pupil scale (m.m.)
- 1
- 2
- 3
- 4
- 5
- 6
- 7
- 8

Blood pressure and Pulse rate

240
230
220
210
200
190
180
170
160
150
140
130
120
110
100
90
80
70
60
50
40
30
Respiration 20
10

Temperature °C
40
39
38
37
36
35
34
33
32
31
30

PUPILS	right	Size		+ reacts − no reaction c. eye closed
		Reaction		
	left	Size		
		Reaction		

L I M B M O V E M E N T	A R M S	Normal power		Record right (R) and left (L) separately if there is a difference between the two sides.
		Mild weakness		
		Severe weakness		
		Spastic flexion		
		Extension		
		No response		
	L E G S	Normal power		
		Mild weakness		
		Severe weakness		
		Extension		
		No response		

Most children feel upset and tearful after a head injury. Not all need to lie down, in fact many are often happier sitting on Mum's lap playing with a toy which should be provided within the department.

If this line of care is undertaken prior to Lisa seeing the doctor, her mother must be re-assured and told that should Lisa become drowsy, more distressed, vomit, or in any way cause concern, they ought to return immediately to the Assessment Area. Should the triage nurse consider it necessary, however, Lisa would rest on a trolley and regular recording of neurological observations be performed. These recordings should be performed by the same nurse on every occasion. When handing the patient over a set of observations should be performed together by both nurses, thus removing the subjective nature of this assessment.

Eye Conditions

Another common condition seen in the assessment area is the eye complaint. Most people will present with a foreign body in their eye, usually a piece of metal, dust or some other fragment from the street or workplace. Occasionally major eye injuries occur, such as chemical or dry burns, intra-orbital or intra-global foreign bodies, severe laceration of the globe or blow out fractures due to a direct blow to the eye.

Other common complaints from patients include the discovery of a subconjunctival haemorrhage without trauma – usually discovered on waking or when a relative or friend mentions the 'blood in the eye'.

Blow out fracture is a fracture of the base of the orbit due to the pressure placed on the eye. The lower part of the eye and inferior rectus muscle is pushed down into this fracture.
Subconjunctival haemorrhage is bleeding either spontaneous or due to trauma from a small capillary under the conjunctiva.

Mr Stephens arrived in the Accident department one morning having noticed a large 'blood shot' eye while shaving. What distressed him was the vivid blood rather than a slight redness and the fact that the blood was in one place while the rest of the globe was white. The nurse assessing Mr Stephens explained that the reason the blood was in one place was due to a small vessel bursting under the conjunctiva.

Subconjunctival haemorrhage

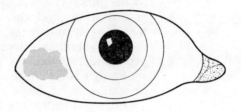

Assessment

A clear history was needed to determine that no trauma had taken place. Severe sneezing, vomiting or coughing may cause this condition due to increased pressure; therefore if the patient gives a history of this it should be noted on the record sheet.

Mr Stephens' visual acuity was investigated. He stood six metres from the eye chart and read the letters from the top down with each eye. The last line able to be read is the visual acuity. In Mr Stephens' case his visual acuity was normal: right 6/6, left 6/6. (The top number represents the six metres from the chart. The lower figure the number of the line read on the chart.)

Because there was no history of trauma, the triage nurse considered other causes of this condition, two possible ones being hypertension or diabetes. With either of these the blood vessels in the eye can be affected and weakened. Spontaneous haemorrhage can occur and this may present as a subconjunctival haemorrhage. Although Mr Stephens gave no history of this, his blood pressure was recorded and blood sugar level obtained by use of a Dextrostix test. (In the majority of cases these tests are normal and no specific cause can be found for the subconjunctival haemorrhage and the patient can be reassured.)

A full assessment of the eye was carried out by the nurse. The eyelids were checked for any encrustation, and the conjunctiva for any foreign body or damage, as was the sclera and globe. The cornea reflected light indicating no oedema due to damage. It was also inspected for foreign bodies. The anterior chamber was present with no blood or foreign body seen. The iris was intact and the pupil central and reactive. From this assessment the nurse was happy that no major condition existed causing need for immediate care, and Mr Stephens could wait until the doctor was free to see him.

The Unwell Child

'I think my baby has had a fit!' This statement usually comes from a very distressed mother, rushing into the Accident & Emergency department with her child lying limp in her arms. The immediate priority is to ensure that the child has a clear airway, that he is breathing and that a carotid pulse is present. These three vital areas of patient care should never be forgotten and must always be assessed before any other injury or condition.

A B C – Airway, Breathing, Circulation

David had all three functioning normally. In fact when the nurse took David he screamed and objected most strongly to being suddenly removed from the comfort of his mother's protective arms. Observing this distress the nurse immediately allowed David's mother to comfort him while obtaining a history of the current problem.

'For the past two days he has been unwell, high temperature and crying when he passes water. This afternoon he appeared warm but shivering, so I wrapped him up well and lit the fire to keep him warm. Suddenly he went stiff, his eyes rolled and he shook all over. He was so hot, I was very frightened, so I called my neighbour and she drove me here.'

This is a typical history of a child suffering a febrile convulsion. Many children when unwell with a high temperature will appear to require added insulation. 'Keep the child warm' is often the instruction mothers are given. Unfortunately, no explanation is provided that by overwrapping the child the temperature will be elevated further; this can lead to the situation that David is now in.

Assessment

Having obtained the history, the triage nurse must now make a full assessment of David. He is crying, so his airway and breathing are both clear. His clothing is removed by his mother to note any rash or infective areas. Body temperature is measured using a rectal thermometer. This gives the most accurate result of core temperature. A urine sample is obtained and tested – protein, blood or any other abnormal finding could indicate the cause of the high temperature, possibly relating to the urinary system. Does the boy look dehydrated, oedematous in any area, especially the eyelids

61

(periorbital oedema)? Is he well nourished? Ask the mother whether there is any family history of 'fits' and if David has any allergies, especially to any antibiotics which might be prescribed later. Having fully assessed David, the doctor would be asked to see him as an urgent priority.

Summary of Walking Patient Assessment

What the case histories on just a few walking patients have attempted to show is that with immediate expert assessment of all those presenting to the Accident & Emergency department, correct nursing care can be given immediately. Patients who should be seen urgently are not left in waiting rooms and those that must wait have been seen and examined prior to that wait.

Without nursing assessment many patients will be denied correct nursing care prior to seeing the doctor; incorrect treatment by friends or relatives will not be discovered and corrected. Patients will not be provided with the care they should expect from a service such as ours.

Also remember, explanation is a key word with assessment. Patients must have the assessment explained to them. If required to wait, this must always be accompanied with the invitation to return to the assessment area should their condition become worse, their wound bleed through the temporary dressing or if they are concerned in any way. With this policy, co-operation will exist between the patient and nursing staff and stress levels on both sides should be reduced.

Nursing on Trolleys/Beds

These patients, unlike the walking patients, will not require an assessment to determine if they can wait in the waiting room; however they still require expert nursing assessment so immediate nursing care can be initiated and priority of care determined. The majority of patients on a stretcher trolley or bed will have been received into the department via the Ambulance Service. They will normally have been conveyed on a stretcher by the ambulance personnel. Some patients may walk into the department or be brought in by use of a chair. In these situations the nurse must assess the patient's requirements and if a stretcher trolley is needed due to the injury or illness, this must be provided.

Needless to say, the types of conditions that patients present with in the Accident Centre are endless. Many will require stretcher or bed care and be admitted to the ward, e.g. acute abdomen, shortness of breath, bleeding per vagina, chest pain, back pain, cerebrovascular accident, multiple injuries. All of them require individual care and the assessment must reflect this.

Cerebrovascular accident is either an embolism, thrombosis or bleed affecting the cerebral flow to the brain. Often a portion of the brain is affected causing loss of function to one side of the body (*hemiparesis*).

Critically Injured Patients

Assessing patients with multiple injuries must be done very rapidly as immediate action is required to prevent further complications. This rapid assessment requires practice, and can be achieved in ninety seconds or less. The priority is to assess the Airway, Breathing and Circulation (A B C):

Airway This must always take priority over all other injuries; without a clear airway a patient will die or receive irreversible brain damage due to inadequate ventilation and gas transfer. A *noisy* airway is an *obstructed* airway. A *quiet* airway *without chest movement* is an *obstructed* airway. A *quiet* airway *with chest movements* is a *clear* airway.

Always check inside the mouth for any blood, vomit, loose teeth or dentures. Gum and boiled sweets are also putting the airway at risk.

Breathing Check to see the chest is moving adequately on inspiration and that the frequency and depth of breathing is sufficient (shallow, rapid or very slow breathing will not allow adequate tidal volume to occur and gas transfer will be impaired). Observe whether both sides of the chest expand on inspiration and that segments of the chest (flail chest) do not move in opposite directions to normal breathing patterns.

Flail chest. Due to injury a segment of chest moves in the opposite direction to chest breathing movements (*paradoxical movement*). This movement occurs when two or more ribs are broken in two or more places.

If you hear air 'sucking' through a wound in the chest, it must be closed immediately (use a pad or even your hand until a secure airtight dressing is available).

Circulation This can be considered in two parts:
1 Cardiac – the pump
2 Vessels and blood – haemorrhage

If the major pulse in the neck (*carotid*) or upper leg/groin (*femoral*) is not present, cardiac arrest has occurred and resuscitation of the heart must commence immediately. Haemorrhage, both internal and external, may be present. The nurse can assess external haemorrhage visually. Blood will be leaving the body via a wound. The blood may be *oozing* out indicating capillary damage, *pouring* out indicating venous damage or *spurting* (like a fountain) indicating arterial damage. Internal haemorrhage is more difficult to observe because, as the name implies, bleeding is taking place inside the body. Assessment of the patient as a whole will present sufficient information to the nurse to assume and deal with internal haemorrhage. The patient will often be pale, the skin moist, and the pulse will be rapid and weak and blood pressure (although not initially) will soon become low. The patient may become restless, complain of thirst and respiration will become rapid. Complaints of feeling cold, despite the warm room, are also a common occurrence – these signs and symptoms are of the condition termed 'shock'.

Having assessed the three major priorities you can now assess the whole patient from head to toe. The scalp, ears, nose and face are checked for any signs of bleeding or other injury. Fluid from the ear may be cerebrospinal fluid (CSF), always consider this possibility. The neck and spinal column are assessed for any damage. Chest and abdomen are observed for any wounds or obvious distension. The pelvis is felt for any fractures and in the male the tip of the meatus is assessed for any blood. (Blood at the tip of the meatus is a sign of possible urethral rupture; should this sign be present, the patient should be encouraged **not** to pass urine. If urine is allowed to leave the bladder it will pass through the rupture into the pelvic cavity.) Arms and legs are checked for movement, colour, warmth, sensation, possible fractures and wounds.

As part of your assessment of the multiply injured patient, property should be checked to identify any medic alert or other means of identifying any underlying allergies or medical condition, e.g. diabetes, drugs that the patient is taking such as steroids. Relatives' phone numbers may be carried; this will aid contacting them.

Clinical observations will be commenced; these will relate to the specific injuries.

Mr Kelly was brought to the Accident Centre after being involved in a road traffic accident. He was a passenger in the front seat of a car which had been hit from the side. The ambulance crew reported to the nurse that after examination their findings were as follows:

Injury to chest

Injury to neck

Injury to pelvis

Injury to upper legs

The history from the driver of the car indicated to the crew that Mr Kelly had not been unconscious at any time since the accident. This history was important because it indicated that the accident had not caused injury to the brain sufficient to cause even a brief lapse of consciousness. A cervical collar had been applied to stabilise any possible neck fracture and to protect the spinal cord from damage. Both legs were splinted to immobilise the evident fractures. This line of care prevents unnecessary movement and further damage of the fracture site and underlying tissues. Oxygen had been administered during the journey to supplement the patient's intake. (Due to the internal haemorrhage oxygen levels in the blood would drop and tissue anoxia would occur.)

It is essential that nurses obtain a complete history and they should always question the ambulance crew for all details of the patient's pre-hospital situation and treatment.

Assessment

NURSING
CARE

Before transfer from the ambulance trolley the nurse performed a rapid assessment of Mr Kelly's injuries so assuring herself that no harm would come to him while being moved onto the department's trolley. Mr Kelly was orientated, able to explain what had happened and obeyed commands; this was established by his conversation with the staff while being transferred to the patient trolley from the ambulance stretcher.

The assessing nurse then began the full assessment of Mr Kelly. It was clear that with conversation in progress his airway was clear and breathing adequate; however one side of his chest was slightly more expanded even on expiration then the other – this sign was immediately reported to the doctor who was in attendance, attempting to site an infusion. Mr Kelly complained of neck pain, pain in the pelvic region and in both legs. The nursing assessment of these areas was undertaken. The neck was gently felt for any abnormal protrusions or wounds. The pelvis was examined for any bruising and the meatus checked for blood. Blood was not present so Mr Kelly was asked to pass urine; this was found to contain microscopic blood, indicating possible damage to the bladder or kidneys.

Both legs were tested for movement of toes and feet. As there was swelling around both thighs with one very deformed, no full leg movements were attempted. Sensation was also checked. Recognising that multiple fractures of the pelvis and femurs were possible, the nurse commenced quarter-hourly observations of pulse, blood pressure and respiration. Any change in these would indicate the extent of internal haemorrhage and the response to treatment. Internal blood loss from fractures of the pelvis and femurs can be as much as 4 to 6 litres.

Observation of respiration was also required frequently as the abnormal chest expansion could indicate a pneumothorax which could suddenly develop into a tension pneumothorax.

The wrist watch which was removed as part of the undressing process and property check

Pneumothorax is air contained in the chest cavity. The air has entered either from damage to the lung or from an outside source i.e. wound in the chest wall.
Tension pneumothorax is a pneumothorax in which the air in the chest cavity is under pressure and if allowed to continue to develop, will cause cardiac and respiratory arrest.

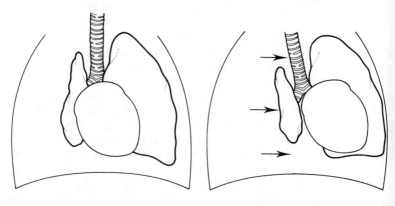

Pneumothorax (left) and tension pneumothorax (right)

was found to contain a medic alert. Details inside indicated that Mr Kelly was allergic to penicillin. It also gave his blood group and his relative's address and telephone number. This information was recorded on his record sheet.

Nursing assessment in this situation had led to correct care being carried out to Mr Kelly's neck, legs and pelvis. The realisation of internal haemorrhage, possible chest trauma and bladder or kidney damage assisted the medical staff in their examination and diagnosis. Without nursing assessment patients would suffer unnecessarily and many signs and symptoms could be missed.

Back Injury

Not all patients on stretchers require admission to hospital; this is often true of back injuries where no bone damage is involved.

HISTORY

John was a forty-five year old builder. He was very fit; he regularly played squash and was active in the local swimming club. On Wednesday afternoon as he was lifting some bricks, his concentration was suddenly broken by a friend calling his name. Without thinking he twisted round and immediately suffered severe pain in his lower back. He was unable to stand and the ambulance was called.

Assessment

On arrival in the department John was in pain; he had been laid flat on the ambulance trolley. Prior to transfer onto the department's trolley the nurse assessed John's injuries. He was then carefully lifted from the ambulance trolley onto a patient care trolley. A scoop stretcher was used for this procedure. The nurse had ascertained from John's immediate needs that he required a trolley where X-rays could be taken without further movements, such as onto an X-ray table. (Not all patient trolleys have this facility.) John gave his history to the nurse before any attempt was made to undress him. This allowed the nurse to establish the exact area of complaint and decide the best method of removing John's clothes. The spine must maintain correct body alignment, and spinal cord damage must be assumed until proven otherwise. Support nurses will be required to help John maintain alignment of his spinal column. Having discovered that the pain was in the lumbar region, the nurse then established sensation and movement in both legs. No neurological damage appeared present, although leg raising was not attempted (leg raising will be painful and should be left to the Medical Officer's examination). Movement of the feet and toes were normal. Feeling of touch was also present.

John was gently undressed with the aid of two nurses. After resting for a short while John was asked to pass urine; he was able to do this so establishing that there was no neurological bladder damage. This nursing assessment here illustrates the need for immediate assessment to ensure that correct facilities and equipment are used and that the subsequent care will not cause further damage. (In some cases of spinal injury clothes may need to be cut. This should only be done if the nursing assessment indicates the need to prevent further damage to the patient's spinal cord.) Using nursing knowledge of spinal injuries, the nurse considered the possible effects to the bladder and asked John to pass urine. John, in fact, had only strained a muscle and was allowed home for bed rest; however, the correct assessment and action on arrival by the nurse would have prevented any further damage had the situation been different, and vertebral fractures or dislocation been present.

Pain Assessment

How each individual reacts to pain will often be determined by the type of pain, area of pain and most important the patient's psychological response to pain. All injuries will cause some pain. Often patients arrive in the A & E department complaining of pain without injury. Chest pain, head pain and abdominal pain are three common complaints. A patient suffering a fractured tibia may complain of some pain especially on movement. Another patient with a similar injury can arrive screaming and crying with pain; how each patient reacts is an individual response.

During your stay in this department you may nurse individuals who are not prescribed analgesic cover despite acute pain. This is normally only withheld in the case of abdominal pain where analgesia would mask signs and symptoms of diagnostic importance for the surgeon. This situation can be very distressing for relatives and nurses within the area. Reassurance and explanation are very important. Surgical staff should see the patient as soon as possible, thus reducing the amount of time the patient must suffer the discomfort.

When assessing the patient's pain you should not only accept what they tell you but look for other indications:

Facial expression

Pulse rate, which will increase with pain

Position of patient, e.g. knees down/up

Protective mechanism (holding the arm, reluctance to be touched)

Screaming and crying are poor indications as much of this can be reactionary.

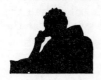

By observing the patient's response to movement and intervention, a much more detailed understanding of their discomfort can be obtained. Remember, many patients will not wish to 'make a fuss' and therefore may suffer with pain in silence. Use your knowledge, physical senses and empathy to help alleviate patient suffering. It is often the nurse who identifies the need for pain relief. Much can be achieved by good nursing care with regard to position and support of limbs and body. Do encourage the medical staff where appropriate to prescribe adequate analgesia, especially where the dressing you are about to perform is likely to cause additional pain. You do not have to use the analgesia if it is not wanted in the event.

Venous or Arterial Obstruction

Assessing patients complaining of possible circulatory obstruction can be difficult. This situation is much worse if information is incorrectly provided by a third person.

HISTORY

Deep vein thrombosis is a thrombus (usually a blood clot) within the lumen of a deep vein; this usually affects the calf veins but is not restricted to this area.

Mrs Thompson had been complaining of pain in her calf muscle for several days. The pain was becoming much worse. The telephone call to the hospital gave the impression that Mrs Thompson was suffering a deep vein thrombosis of her left leg. The medical team on call had agreed to accept this patient for treatment.

Assessment

NURSING CARE

Arterial embolism is an embolism (usually a moving blood clot) which travels in the circulating system and if within the arterial system will cause an obstruction to blood flow.

On arrival the nurse took a history from Mrs Thompson and then assessed her leg. On comparison the left leg was much paler than the right. There was no obvious swelling at the calf. No peripheral pulses could be felt in the lower leg and the skin was extremely cold. The nurse immediately contacted the doctor indicating the possibility not of a deep vein thrombosis but of an arterial embolism. This was found to be correct and immediate referral to surgical colleagues resulted in Mrs Thompson being taken to the operating theatre rapidly.

This illustrates the need for a thorough nursing assessment even though a provisional diagnosis may have been made by a third party. Once the patient arrives in the department it is our responsibility to undertake this assessment and prevent the correct treatment being delayed. Had Mrs Thompson had a swollen, hot, painful leg, it is possible she would have been suffering a deep vein thrombosis. Some delay if necessary before seeing the doctor could have been acceptable. With an arterial embolism no delay was acceptable and rather than Urgent priority, Mrs Thompson was rated as Immediate priority.

Fred – the tramp

'We've got Fred in the ambulance, which cubicle would you like him in?'

This statement, and question, brought a smile to the triage nurse's face. Fred was a local tramp and every Tuesday he would 'collapse' in the town centre knowing that he would receive a bath and supper in hospital before being sent on his way. He always complained of some chest pain and feeling dizzy.

This type of patient can be mishandled if the nurses and medical staff become complacent with a 'regular attender'. The nurse must always undertake a full assessment irrespective of the regular frequency of the complaint. Just because Fred always complains of chest pain, it does not mean that today he is not suffering a myocardial infarction.

Assessment

Fred – like all patients – was undressed and clinical observation recorded. In addition to pulse, blood pressure, temperature and respiration, Dextrostix and ECG was performed. The general unkempt condition of Fred was noted and his undernourished, dehydrated body observed. No specific reason could be found for his chest pain or dizziness today but that normal glint in Fred's eye was missing. The triage nurse had seen Fred too often, she knew that something was wrong.

'It's at night,' Fred said, 'I just can't get my breath, been like it for two days now. When I cough there is blood coming up.' The triage nurse immediately reported this to the doctor who undertook further investigations and Fred was admitted.

Summary

In this chapter we have discussed the assessment of patients by nurses. Both walking and stretcher patients require assessment on admission. Assessing a patient is a team responsibility, it should not be left to a doctor or nurse but performed by both at varying times.

Airway, breathing, circulation – this order of priority must always be maintained. Assessing a patient goes further than the clinical observation of the condition or injury. It must include psychological and social needs and should include where possible the relatives and friends of the patient. We must never forget each patient is a person, each person is an individual.

5   Identifying Actual and Potential Problems

Information gathered in the assessment stage can now be sorted and analysed. This allows the nurse to identify actual and potential problems. Problems should also be put in order of importance. An actual obstructed airway takes priority over the potential fractured femur. Patients may have clearly defined evident (*actual*) problems; many may also have problems that can arise (*potential*) if correct nursing intervention is not carried out. When identifying patients' problems it is important to include both actual and potential problems.

Examples of actual (A) and potential (P) problems:

1   Francesca is unable to stand without assistance (A) and may fall if left alone (P).
2   Mrs Brown has swelling of her hand due to trauma (A) and blood flow in her third finger may be reduced if the ring becomes tight (P).
3   Gary has a pain in his neck due to injury (A) and the spinal cord may be damaged if incorrectly handled (P).

With nearly all patients seen in the department a potential problem can exist. For example, patients presenting with a wound will be asked about their tetanus cover. The wound is visible, it is an actual problem. Tetanus infection is a potential problem of having a wound. By identifying if tetanus immunity has been provided at an earlier stage in the patient's life, the nurse is also assessing the potential risk to the patient. If the patient has

Tetanus is an infection caused by *Clostridium tetani*, via a contaminated wound. *Clostridium tetani* is found in soil and manure, therefore any wound may be susceptible to infection, especially deep wounds e.g. puncture wounds or wounds with a poor blood supply. Prevention is by active immunity (a toxin is given and the individual produces antibodies). If protection has not been undertaken before the wound occurs, positive immunity can be made available e.g. Humotet (antibodies injected directly into patient).

been immunised at some stage, the risk of infection is lower than if no immunity had ever been obtained.

Potential problems may not necessarily relate directly to the patient's presenting condition, they may appear after treatment in the department. For example, patients given an anaesthetic for reduction of a fracture have the potential risk of airway obstruction; the potential problem has thus been created within the A & E Unit. Wang Lee has a swollen, deformed wrist (A), pain in his wrist (A) and may have impaired blood flow to the hand (P). X-ray examination shows a fractured radius (A). Reduction is required; this treatment generates potential problems that did not exist earlier:

May have obstructed airway (P)
May vomit under anaesthetic (P)
May react adversely to anaesthetic (P)
Plaster of Paris may become tight(P)

Actual problems are not always easy to identify. It often requires the skill of a trained nurse with experience in Accident and Emergency nursing. The ambulance crew on arrival with a patient in cardiac arrest comments on the difficulty inflating the lungs (A); that the chest appears over-inflated on one side – increased size of chest mainly on one side (A); and that the carotid pulse is poorly felt during cardiac massage – poor arterial perfusion (A). History and signs tell the experienced nurse that a tension pneumothorax is present (A) and immediate intervention is required.

Although this was an actual problem it might not have been identified by a less experienced person. This is in contrast to, say, a foreign body sitting on the cornea of the eye. The foreign body can be clearly seen, and no damage to the eye has occurred other than that caused by the foreign body. In this situation the actual problem is obvious: foreign body on the cornea of the eye (A).

Because of the nature of the work and intervention required, nursing problems and medical diagnosis often become interrelated. The nurse must identify nursing problems that doctors will not consider and also the nursing intervention will be concerned with the presenting problem and not necessarily the diagnosis. For example, a patient is brought to the department unconscious. The medical diagnosis will determine the subsequent treatment; the actual problem however on admission is an unconscious patient. Nursing intervention involves implementing correct positioning, nursing care, obtaining a clear history from ambulance staff, identifying the patient, contacting relatives. The nurse will also help the medical staff obtain a diagnosis by carrying out specific investigations such as head to toe examination, pulse, blood pressure, temperature, Dextrostix (BM Stix) and electrocardiograph tracing. For the unconscious patient various potential problems can also be highlighted:

Unconscious patient (A)
Airway obstruction (P)
Impaired breathing (P)
Pressure sores if not turned (P)
Incontinence/retention of urine (P)

Many more potential problems must be considered by ward nursing staff such as diet, fluids and limb movement. The A & E nurse is interested in potential problems that may require intervention while the patient is in the department. Because the nurse identifies potential problems that can influence medical diagnosis, the relationship between medical and nursing staff must always be one of close harmony in the working environment.

The nurse, after ensuring correct positioning and airway care of the unconscious patient, commences investigations. One reason for a patient becoming unconscious is low blood sugar (*hypoglycaemia*) in someone suffering from diabetes. The Dextrostix (BM Stix) test will show this level (normal blood sugar level is 2.5–4.7 mmol/l). The medical officer can then diagnose the cause, and medical treatment can be administered. In A & E the line between nursing and medical problems is thin, however it must remain.

Another example of where nursing problems and the medical diagnosis will be recorded in a different manner is with a patient with respiratory difficulty. The problems for the nurse to identify and deal with may be:

Shortness of breath (A)
Difficulty in maintaining upright position in bed (A)
Difficulty with expectoration of sputum (A)
Fear and the feeling of drowning (A)

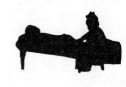

The doctor may diagnose a chest infection or pulmonary oedema; he will then prescribe specific treatment. Nursing problems will still exist and correct nursing intervention still be required.

Many patients in Accident and Emergency will have problems that, although identified by nursing staff, will require intervention not from nursing but from another source.

Good nursing care involves identifying all the patient's actual and potential problems; many may develop after the patient returns home. The nurse who assessed Mrs James (the lady with a wrist injury) identified these potential problems after discharge:

Wrist injury (A)
Will require plaster of Paris (P)
Inability to undertake housework (P)
Inability to cook meals (P)
Inability to wash/bathe (P)

The social workers and district nurses will need to be involved if no relatives can help cope with these problems. Nursing staff in A & E cannot alleviate the problems which may become actual problems once the patient arrives home; the nurse must refer to other health care teams in the hospital and becomes for a short time co-ordinator of the patient's care.

6 Goal Setting and Nurse Intervention

Nurse intervention can take many forms. It does not necessarily have to relate directly to the patient. Nurse intervention in A & E may be totally occupied with helping the relatives or friends of patients who have died or been brought in dead.

Intervention may involve dealing with violent or potentially violent patients, attempting to control a drunken individual or preventing a depressed patient committing suicide. It may include assisting a mother and child over the physical and psychological trauma of suturing the child's wound. It implies taking action at each extreme of care, from a grazed knee to a cardiac arrest.

Every caring situation must have a goal for which to aim. It may be that the goal is to prevent the violent patient smashing the window. It may be stemming the flow of the blood from a wound. It may be the reduction of pain from a fracture. Whatever the goal there will always be many ways to achieve it.

Stemming the flow of blood from a wound can take various types of intervention. It will include pressure and elevation. It may require varied pressure according to the type of wound; the way pressure is applied will depend on the presence or absence of a foreign body. The use of elevation depends on the area of the wound and whether a fracture is or is not present. The nurse must, after assessment and problem identification, decide on the goal of care and then take appropriate action to achieve that goal.

Goals in the department should be practical and may be short term. It is useless creating goals that are impossible to achieve, e.g. a patient with chronic respiratory disorder will not benefit from a goal aiming at normal ventilation. A goal of improved respiratory function may however be achieved, and appropriate action by the nurse can result in this goal being met. Long term goals are important and necessary but often will not be totally achieved by the nurses in the department. Nurse intervention in alliance with medical action provides care for the patient. It is important to always consider intervention in A & E as a team approach.

Many patients require immediate action by nurses before medical intervention. Chapter Four dealt with assessment. Immediately after this stage of patient care nursing intervention is required. Most patients must wait to see the doctor; sometimes this may be hours rather than minutes. During this period nurse intervention can do much to aid the patient and make the wait as comfortable and risk free as possible. Ice packs applied to swollen limbs, slings to injured arms, temporary dressings to wounds, are all examples of intervention.

The A, B, C of Care

Just as you remember the first three letters of the alphabet, you should also remember the priority of patient care – A, B, C:

Airway
Breathing
Circulation

When dealing with any patient always ask yourself three questions:

1 Is the patient's airway clear?
2 Is the patient breathing adequately?

3 Is the patient's heart beating and blood remaining within the circulation?

If any answers are 'No', then immediate intervention is required.

A – Airway: If not clear it must be made clear – How?

1 *Position* – when possible always nurse patients on their side; this prevents fluid trickling down the trachea and helps the tongue remain clear of the oral pharynx.

2 *Jaw movement* – always bring the jaw forward; this pulls the tongue away from the oral pharynx.

3 *Suction* – good oral suction using high powered suction equipment will remove vomit, saliva and other fluids which can cause airway obstruction.

4 *Guedal airway* – this will help prevent the tongue falling back into the oral pharynx; it does not replace correct positioning of patient.

A Guedal airway is a rubber or other material instrument that will sit in the oropharyngeal area and assist in establishing a clear airway by supporting the tongue.

The upper airway

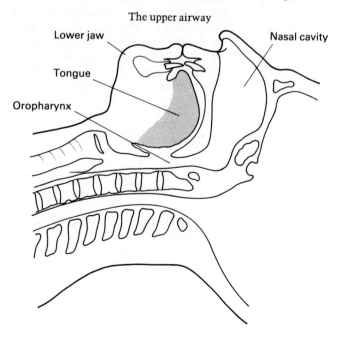

Lower jaw

Nasal cavity

Tongue

Oropharynx

B – Breathing: If not breathing, you must intervene – How?

1 Clear airway as above.

2 Perform positive pressure ventilation (mouth to mouth resuscitation or use bag and mask with oxygen attached).

C – Circulation: If the patient's heart is not beating, intervene – How?

1 Perform closed cardiac massage.

If blood is being lost from the system, prevent this – How?

1 Pressure on the point of bleeding.

2 Elevation of bleeding point to slow blood flow.

Nurse intervention in one or all three areas is the most important life saving action you will ever take. Remember – A,B,C.

Cardiac Arrest

This is possibly one of the most alarming situations learners find themselves dealing with. Cardiac arrest can occur due to cardiac related conditions, to a neurological or hypovolaemic state. Although the immediate resuscitation remains the same, subsequent treatment to restore circulation will depend on the cause. For example, replacement of lost fluid and prevention of further haemorrhage is the treatment for cardiac arrest related to hypovolaemia. Cardiac arrest due to abnormalities within the electrical conductor of the heart are treated in various ways, with drugs and electrical defibrillation being the most common methods. The most common cardiac related problems are either sudden unexplained ventricular fibrillation, asystole or myocardial infarction. Studies in Seattle, USA, suggest that only 20 per cent of cardiac related sudden deaths are due to acute infarction.

Hypovolaemia is a loss of body fluid due to blood or plasma loss (a decrease from the normal volume).
Ventricular fibrillation is unco-ordinated activity within the ventricular myocardium. It causes failure of cardiac output and shows on a cardiac monitor as an irregular unco-ordinated wave.

Patients suffering cardiac arrest within the A & E department have a good prognosis, but it depends very much on the immediate intervention of the nursing staff. The goals are:

1 Provide the patient with assisted ventilation.

2 Provide the patient with assisted cardiac function.

These goals are achieved by cardiopulmonary resuscitation (CPR).

This action by the nurse must continue until normal physiology returns or the medical staff consider the goal of survival unachievable. For the nurse to be able to intervene an assessment must be made and problems identified. Assessment will be of a patient suddenly collapsed – unconscious:

Cyanosis is a blue/black appearance of the skin due to a lack of oxygen in the circulation.

The skin will be pale or cyanosed.

Normal breathing will be absent.

Major pulses in the neck (carotid) or groin (femoral) will be absent.

The nurse must intervene at once. The brain will only survive for two to three minutes; oxygen must be received and the only way this can occur is by pushing oxygen into the lungs under pressure. The heart must be massaged to stimulate cardiac activity and maintain circulation throughout the body until normal cardiac output returns.

In resuscitation areas of an A & E department, resuscitation bags and masks will be present. Oxygen should be attached to this bag and the mask placed over the patient's mouth and nose. Squeezing the bag pushes air under pressure into the patient's lungs. If these bags are not available, mouth to mouth ventilation must take place.

Cardiac massage is achieved by placing the heel of one hand over the lower half of the sternum and using the other hand on top of the first, compress the sternum 1½ to 2 in (4 to 5 cm). Use fifteen compressions and two ventilations. If two people are available use five compressions to one ventilation. The following table is a quick guide to nurse intervention during a cardiac arrest:

Assess that arrest is present.
Summon help – alarm bell or shout.
Place patient flat on a firm surface, establish a clear airway.
Inflate the lungs, four inflations rapidly.
Check carotid pulse.
Commence cardiac massage, 15 compressions.
Inflate the lungs, two inflations.
Continue 15 and 2 until help arrives, then 5 and 1 (recommended ratio by the British Resuscitation Council).
Second person arriving sends for Casualty Officer and Arrest Team.

HISTORY

When Mr Simpson suffered a cardiac arrest the learners knew exactly what to do. While the staff nurse was clearing the patient's airway and starting ventilation, one learner was assisting the circulation with external cardiac massage.

The other learners in the resuscitation room were aware that on the arrival of the doctors advanced life support equipment would be required. This was prepared:

1   Intravenous infusion of either dextrose 5 per cent or sodium bicarbonate 8.4 per cent
2   Intravenous drugs
3   Monitor/defibrillator
4   Equipment for intubation

Intubation (endotracheal) is the insertion of a tube into the trachea. Allows for ventilation to the lungs without loss of air and oxygen to the stomach.

The preparation and checking of drugs was left to a trained member of staff but the nurse learners assisted the doctors while siting the infusion and carrying out intubation. One learner knew the correct position of the monitor leads so this speeded up the procedure of identifying the arrhythmia present.

While this resuscitation continued Mrs Simpson was taken to the relatives' room and given a cup of tea. She will always remember the help that the nurse gave her, saying that just being with someone helped. Intervention is not always related to the patient, it is often with the care and support provided to relatives and friends that nurses can do so much to help.

Many cardiac arrests with which you may cope during your stay in A & E will occur in the pre-hospital setting. Relatives often give a history of the patient's sudden collapse either in the house or street. Resuscitation by the public often is not attempted or incorrectly applied. Although ambulance crews will attempt resuscitation during the journey to hospital, several minutes have elapsed before their arrival at the scene. Because of this many patients in cardiac arrest arriving in A & E will not survive. This should not prevent any attempt at resuscitation by departmental staff and should not encourage the learner to misinterpret the success rate of cardiac arrest generally.

The Multiply Injured Patient

This patient's life is in your hands. Incorrect care or lack of intervention will result in either death, further disability or irreversible damage to the brain or spinal cord.

HISTORY

Mr Kelly you will recall had suffered injury to his chest, neck, pelvis and upper legs. Fortunately he was orientated to time and place (which indicates that there is no serious head injury and he can attend to his own airway) and although in severe hypovolaemic shock, was able to participate in his care. Movement was restricted so all clothes were cut off and bagged following checks for property. No clothing should be thrown away. It is useful as a clue for the police and still belongs personally to Mr Kelly who is the only one who can decide to throw it out. The A, B, C of care was carried out:

Airway: This was clear and conversation was taking place.

Breathing: This was difficult due to the chest injury; tidal volume level was acceptable but oxygen was given to supplement the room air. Following medical examination a right sided haemopneumothorax was diagnosed. A chest drain was inserted by the doctor to relieve this condition and connected to an underwater seal drain. (Removal of blood and air from the chest is achieved by inserting a drain into the chest cavity. Ventilation of the lung can then be achieved and tidal volume will increase. Prevention of re-entry of air is

Tidal volume is the amount of air which passes in and out of the lungs during normal respiratory action. **Haemopneumothorax means** both blood and air are within the chest cavity due to chest trauma.

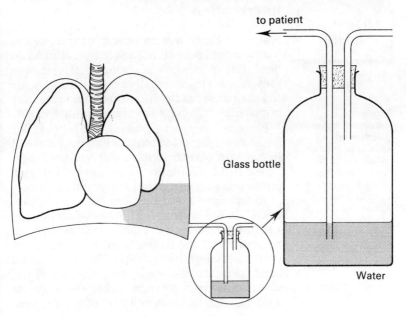

to patient

Glass bottle

Water

achieved by connecting the drain to an under-water seal system, as this only permits one way movement of air.)

Circulation: This was grossly inadequate due to the loss of blood from internal injuries. Blood had escaped from vessels in the chest, pelvis and legs. Rapid pulse and low blood pressure reflected the situation, as did the cold clammy skin (peripheral shutdown of skin vessels).

Intravenous replacement of blood was needed; however first his blood must be cross-matched and grouped by sending blood samples to the laboratory. During this waiting period the blood volume will be increased with a volume expander. The most common solution used in this situation is Haemaccel. Large bore cannuli were inserted in both arm veins and infusion commenced rapidly.

Haemaccel is a synthetic blood replacement fluid used where blood volume or plasma volume replacement is required.

Intervention

NURSING
CARE

Pain: Mr Kelly was in severe pain from the fractures and general trauma to his body. As no head injury existed a strong analgesic was prescribed. This is usually given intravenously in small doses as the intramuscular route may not be effective due to peripheral shutdown.

Peripheral shutdown means that venous and arterial circulation within the skin is diminished. The skin becomes cold and pale. It is difficult to cannulate veins.

Fracture support: Having stabilised Mr Kelly's breathing and circulation, the next step in his care was to support the fractured legs. These had been supported on the trolley with pillows during the initial resuscitation procedure and now could be more adequately controlled in leg splints. A Thomas splint or Trac 3 splint can be used to enable fixed traction to be applied to the limbs. Care must be taken when applying these splints. Traction must be maintained on the leg by one member of the team, holding it straight while the splint is applied. Skin traction or a heel support is then fixed to the limb and traction applied from the splint.

Thomas splint

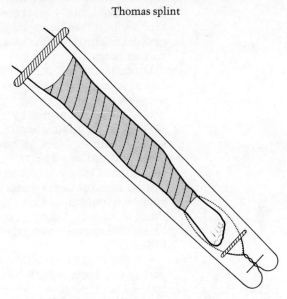

Catheterisation is normally carried out in patients suffering injuries such as this, but Mr Kelly passed urine voluntarily. A decision as to the need for urethral catheterisation depends on the requirement for accurate urinary measurement, the patient's general condition, and his ability to pass urine adequately.

X-rays of the neck, chest, pelvis and both femurs will be ordered by the doctor in charge. Results of these X-rays showed no fracture to the cervical spine, though the cervical collar was maintained because of the pain in the neck. Several ribs were fractured. The right lung was now more expanded, while the left lung was normal. The pelvis was fractured across the ileum. Both femurs were fractured mid shaft.

Nursing observations continued throughout the time spent in the resuscitation room and these improved gradually. When available blood was commenced after the nurse checked carefully that the bag corresponded with all details available, e.g. record number, name, blood group, bag number, date issued and expiry date. The first unit was given rapidly over half an hour.

During all this time Mrs Kelly was contacted and then supported with regular updates by the nursing staff.

Goals had been met by the time Mr Kelly was ready for main theatre. Intervention had stabilised him. Now he could have his fractures reduced, skeletal traction applied and be sent to the Orthopaedic ward from theatre.

Intervention is very much a team effort in such a situation as this. Nurses and doctors must work in harmony. A team leader needs to be identified and instruction from this person followed.

It is difficult to separate nursing and medical care in the acute stages; however, nurses have specific duties both before the arrival and during the care of the patient.

Before arrival: All equipment must be prepared within the resuscitation area.

Intravenous infusion run through giving sets. Packs open to allow procedures, such as cut down, underwater seal drainage and peritoneal lavage. Equipment for collecting blood for crossmatch and grouping.

Intubation equipment.

Oxygen must be turned on, suction at the ready.

Records and observation charts.

X-ray informed of pending arrival.

Medical staff prepared to receive patient.

On arrival: Nurses must assess the patient before moving him from the ambulance trolley to the department's stretcher care trolley. Airway must be assessed and intervention car-

Cut down – due to peripheral shutdown the veins may need exposure by a small surgical incision to allow for cannulation.

ried out. In Mr Kelly's case intervention here was not required as assessment indicated a clear airway and he was conscious.

Oxygen was administered as soon as Mr Kelly was placed on the trolley. A cervical neck collar applied. His clothes were cut off rather than removed normally to prevent any further movement of the limbs. It is also important to maintain his dignity, so cover him up as soon as possible with a blanket.

Having assessed breathing and the over-expansion of the right chest, underwater seal drainage was prepared and assistance was given to the medical staff. Observation of the drain once inserted becomes a nursing responsibility and the nurse must note the amount of drainage and 'swing' of fluid in the tube. All drainage must be recorded on a fluid chart. Excess drainage other than the initial blood loss from the chest must be reported to the doctor at once as this could indicate continuous bleeding within the chest. The 'swing' of water in the tube indicates that drainage is progressing properly. If this stops report to the medical staff.

Because of shock and his low blood pressure, Mr Kelly remained lying flat. Quarter-hourly recording of pulse and blood pressure measured the response to treatment. Internal haemorrhage was controlled by moving the patient as little as possible and replacing lost fluid with a high molecular substance (Haemaccel). Nurses assisted with this procedure and monitored fluid intake via this route.

All procedures were explained and continuous reassurance was given by nurses at the head of the trolley. Nothing is worse than trying to give reassurance from the foot end of the trolley.

The amount of urine passed was measured and recorded. This provided an accurate method of determining the blood flow and blood pressure within the kidneys.

Giving information and reassurance to relatives and friends is also a nursing duty which must be maintained.

Note: Had Mr Kelly suffered wounds to the skin, these would have been dressed, and tetanus toxoid and antibiotics given if required. It was noticed that Mr Kelly was allergic to penicillin so other forms of antibiotic care would have been used.

Burns and Scald Injury

Burns are dry injuries to the skin. They can result from several sources: excessive heat, such as a naked flame, chemical substances, electrical currents and intense cold. Scalds are wet injuries due to hot liquid, such as boiling water or steam. The depth and degree of burn will determine the course of events, e.g. a superficial burn to a hand or arm will not normally warrant admission to hospital, a 25–40 per cent burn would need to be dealt with much more dramatically, requiring intravenous replacement of fluid and admission to a Burns Unit. Many patients are able to be discharged after treatment in the A & E department. Age is a very important factor when considering admission or outpatient care. A burn on a child can cause many more problems than a similar injury to an adult.

The depth of a burn or scald is described as superficial or deep. Superficial can vary from mild reddening of the skin to blistering and fluid loss from the area of damage. Deep burns totally destroy the skin and subcutaneous tissue and can involve nerve and muscle layers going down to bone.

Any burns or scalds involving the patient's face or neck can affect the airway and respiratory obstruction should always be considered a possibility.

The degree of burn area is mapped using one of many scales devised to estimate area affected and fluid replacement required. Wallace's rule of nine is often used to estimate rapidly the area affected. The body surface is divided into percentage areas. The burned areas are added together and a total area of damage can be estimated. Other scales can be

Wallace's rule of nine

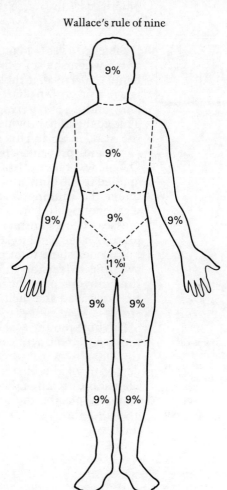

used to arrive at a more precise percentage o
damage.

Each department can vary in the type o
dressing applied to the patient's burn; some
use a vaseline gauze dressing, others various
antibiotic creams. The one major issue is
potential infection; burns can be easily in
fected and strict aseptic technique must be
practised by the nurse when carrying out such
a dressing.

HISTORY

Debbie, a 26 year old model, was making a cup
of tea when she spilt the boiling water on her
hand. On arrival at the A & E department the
triage nurse immediately identified the prob
lem, and a short term goal was established
This goal was to provide immediate cooling to
the scalded area. This reduces heat, relieves
pain and prevents further tissue damage
Debbie was taken into a cubicle and cold water
applied to the burn simply by putting her hand
under the running cold tap. While the hand
was cooling the nurse prepared cold com
presses using normal saline. These were
placed on the hand to keep it cool.

Another short term goal was prevention o
swelling by raising the hand high to reduce
fluid movement to the injured site. Rings were
first removed and then the hand elevated in a
sling.

Having seen the scald, the Casualty Officer
prescribed treatment consisting of deroofing o
the blister on the second and third finger
deroofing of the blister on the back of hand
Flamazine cream and gauze dressing. (Flama
zine and placing the hand in a plastic bag is
also a method of treatment favoured by some
doctors.)

Deroofing is the
removal of the
complete covering
of skin, usually
applied to the
removal of skin
holding fluid from
a burn (*blister*).

The long term goals were:

1 Complete healing of the wound
2 Prevention of infection
3 Return to normal function of the hand

To achieve these goals requires expert nursing care, aseptic technique and time. Rushing a burns dressing can lead to dead tissue being left in the wound and thus possible infection.

NURSING CARE

Intervention

Debbie's hand was cleaned with normal saline. Using sterile scissors and forceps the blisters were deroofed, as this allows for healing without further accumulation of fluid under the skin layer. Flamazine cream was applied to the wound and then gauze over this. Each finger was dressed individually to prevent adhesions between them developing as the healing process took place. A gauze bandage was applied to hold the dressing in place. Subsequent dressings were put on after three days and as necessary during the healing period. On each visit the dressing was performed by a nurse.

This case history shows how nursing intervention is important both before and after the patient sees the doctor. Short and long term goals can be achieved as the patient was treated by the A & E department as an outpatient.

The Fractured Limb

A fracture is a break in the continuity of a bone. This is normally associated with trauma, but on occasions can be due to underlying pathology. The patient will usually complain of pain at the site of the injury and swelling and deformity are often present. Having assessed the limb and identified the problem, action must now be taken. The goal is prevention of movement of the fracture site. By achieving this goal other goals are also achieved, such as reduction in pain, prevention of possible complications, e.g. nerve or blood vessel damage from the fractured bone, and reduction of blood loss (internal) at the fracture site.

Movement of fractured bones is best prevented by the use of splintage. There are various types of splints in the A & E department and you will be shown the correct use and application of each.

Fractured tibia is a common injury sustained on the football field. 'I heard a loud crack as I went down,' is often the history given by the young enthusiast arriving in the department on a wintery Sunday morning. This fracture can cause a great deal of pain and distress. Little support from muscle is afforded to this bone, thus the fracture site tends to be very unstable. Soft tissue can become interposed between the bone ends and healing is restricted.

Many patients may arrive with some form of splintage already on the leg. This may need to be removed for a complete assessment of the limb. Care must be taken when removing the splint and there should be no sudden movements.

Resplintage is important at this stage of care. Slight elevation of the leg once splinted will help reduce swelling. With the fracture site supported and the leg elevated, pain will be less severe and internal bleeding reduced. The goals will have been achieved. Analgesia will also be prescribed by the doctor and is given intramuscularly.

Nursing action must include regular checks on circulation to the limb. An X-ray will outline the fracture and thus aid reduction. Reduction of the tibia can be difficult and skeletal traction may be required. Reduction of a Colles fracture of the wrist usually proves much easier and the patient can return home that day.

HISTORY

You will recall Mrs James, the seventy year old lady who fell injuring her wrist. The triage nurse intervened by placing the arm in a broad sling to support the injury. After an X-ray and diagnosis of a fracture, arrangements were made for Mrs James to have closed reduction under general anaesthetic. This procedure was explained to Mrs James and her consent obtained. Preparation prior to and care during the procedure is very much a nurse's responsibility. Goals can be seen to be different with the various members of the team. The goal of the Casualty Officer is to realign the fractured bones to the best position possible. The goal of the plaster technician is to apply a plaster of Paris cast to support the reduced fracture. The anaesthetist has a goal of maintaining anaesthesia and airway control. The nurse's goal must be to protect the patient from harm, ensuring that all preparation is correct, equipment is functioning and maintaining patient dignity during anaesthesia. Mrs James, when lying on the operating table, must be correctly supported. Arms and legs must not be allowed to fall or sustain abnormal pressure.

As a learner in the A & E department you will have the opportunity of observing a reduction of fracture.

Intervention

Prepare Mrs James by undressing her (including removal of jewellery and dentures) and helping her into a gown and then recording her pulse and blood pressure. Possibly an ECG will be ordered due to her age. Preparation also involves explaining that she will be 'put to sleep, her arm straightened and then a plaster of Paris cast applied'. At any age the fear of anaesthesia is always present; at seventy years of age many patients are very nervous. You can help Mrs James a great deal by spending some time just talking and reassuring her. If you are going to be present during the reduction tell her this. It is always reassuring to a patient to know that a familiar nurse will be there throughout.

General anaesthetic is not always used. Local anaesthetic blocks are quite commonly used (e.g. Biers block).

Once the reduction was complete and anaesthesia discontinued, Mrs James was turned onto her side. This allows control of the airway. Also if vomiting were to occur it would drain from her mouth, not down her throat or airway. A Guedal airway was in situ; this helps to support the tongue from moving back into the oral pharynx and obstructing the airway passages. Suction equipment was readily available should this be required to remove excess saliva. The trained nurse explained that every respiration should be effortless with the chest expanding. Air should be felt on the hand as expiration takes place. Breathing should be quiet indicating a clear airway.

After the reduction the trained nurse remained with Mrs James until she woke from the anaesthesia. This gives you the opportunity to observe airway care of the unconscious patient.

As Mrs James recovered she expelled the

Anaesthetic (local) is a chemical substance which blocks sensory nerve conduction and thus prevents pain being felt distal to the administration site. With the use of a tourniquet local anaesthetic can be injected into the venous system of a limb and this will block sensory conduction of the limb by absorption into the tissues directly from the circulatory system.

Guedal airway and became rousable. Once fully awake she was allowed to rest until the doctor approved her discharge. The arm, now in a plaster of Paris cast, was supported in a sling, and circulation to the fingers was observed. Discharge advice was given.

Nurse intervention with patients suffering from fractures can be seen to be vital to the outcome. Incorrect care on arrival can lead to further damage at the fracture site, increased pain and poor healing. Care throughout the reduction and afterwards is essential; the patient has been placed in a very vulnerable state, and nurse intervention must ensure the patient is protected at all times.

A Patient with a Minor Wound

Many minor wounds affecting only the superficial layer of the skin can be closed adequately with the use of steristrip skin closures. This procedure is carried out by the nursing staff and can easily be undertaken by the learner after instruction and supervised practice. The important thing to always remember is never to exert tension on the skin; the wound edges should always be brought together and the steristrip applied over the closed wound.

HISTORY

Mrs Briggs had been cutting some meat when the knife slipped and cut her finger. Although it bled quite profusely at first, by the time she was seen by the doctor, the wound only required closure with four or five steristrips. Mrs Briggs last had a tetanus course eight years ago, so a booster injection of tetanus toxoid was also prescribed.

Intervention

The nurse undertaking the treatment explained to Mrs Briggs that the wound would be cleaned and 'paper stitches' applied. Using aseptic technique she cleaned the wound and after drying it drew the skin edges together. Steristrips were applied and a gauze dressing put over these. Mrs Briggs was advised not to allow the wound to become wet. She was told that she could remove the dressing and steristrips in one week's time, but if she had any problems or difficulties she could return.

The tetanus toxoid booster injection was drawn up and checked with another nurse. Mrs Briggs was asked if any allergic or local reaction had ever taken place with previous injections. She replied in the negative. The nurse then injected the booster using a deep subcutaneous route at the top of the arm.

Many injuries presenting in the A & E department can be dealt with in this manner; again the amount of nursing action in patient care is evidently great – the whole treatment is undertaken by the nurse.

The Dirty Wound

Having come from the ward environment to A & E, you may find the method of cleaning a wound changes. Wounds, especially on the Surgical ward, are clean and require a straight sweeping action when cleaned. Using a cotton wool ball, the wound is wiped with little pressure and only once per swab.

Dirty wounds in A & E need much more vigorous cleaning. Use of a soapy solution helps remove the dirt from wounds such as grazed knees from the gravel playground. If these wounds need scrubbing a local anaesthetic may be required. This will be administered by the doctor but wound toilet will normally be conducted by the nurse.

Using a sterile brush the wound is gently scrubbed to remove all dirt and gravel. Good circular cleaning with gauze swabs after this will remove all contamination. Use of forceps for this procedure is often inappropriate; however, with the nurse wearing sterile gloves and using sterile equipment, the procedure remains aseptic.

If the patient does not have immunity against tetanus, a course of tetanus immunisation should be commenced. Immediate protection can be provided by the administration of tetanus antibodies (usually Humotet 250 iu intramuscular).

The Patient who has taken an overdose

Some patients arrive with a history of taking an excess amount of tablets. The reasons for this are varied and nursing action must not only deal with the physical removal of the tablets from the body but the psychological help that these patients will need to identify their problem.

HISTORY

Nurse learners may not always feel their intervention is appropriate; however, had it not been for the learner in this department last year a middle aged man may not be settled today. Mr Kemp arrived with his wife. He had taken twenty paracetamol tablets half an hour before his arrival. Mr Kemp refused a stomach lavage or the administration of an emetic. 'I did not want to come here, it was my wife who brought me.' The nurse learner listened with interest. She asked Mr Kemp how his wife, a small lady, was able to bring him to the department if he really did not want help. Seeing an obvious rapport developing, the trained nurse left the cubicle and allowed the learner to continue. The two spoke for some time, not about treatment but about why he felt the need to take the tablets. Many problems were identified, most of which the nurse could not resolve but she did explain the help available through the Psychiatric department and other official bodies. The nurse learner appeared from inside the cubicle and told the doctor that Mr Kemp would now consent to treatment.

Nurse intervention here had helped save a life, not necessarily because it would have been lost due to the overdose, but because it might have lost its quality. This intervention was just as important as the intervention required by a patient with multiple injuries or cardiac arrest.

A Frightened Child

With most children the thought of sutures creates a frightened tearful individual. Mother puts on a brave face and tells the child it will not hurt, she herself being apprehensive about the whole situation and still shaking from the child's injury.

Nursing intervention can help the situation, by talking, explaining and becoming the patient's advocate. The nurse can create a bond between herself and the mother and child by correctly handling the child and helping the mother to cope with her worries. Mum will want to stay with the child yet be concerned that she will be in the way. Correct preparation and positioning of both mother and child will prevent this problem.

Stephen was five years of age. He had just started school and felt very proud that he was growing up. When he cut his leg and required sutures this brave young man suddenly was not as grown up as he thought. He was frightened and soon let us all know with his crying and holding on to his mother.

Intervention

Upon entering the suture room, he became interested in the toys and the pictures on the wall. Knowing that 'Basil Brush' was watching over him stemmed the tears. Mother helped to wrap him in a blanket, leaving one arm free for her to hold. She was positioned at the head of the trolley, where she could talk and reassure Stephen while the suturing was carried out. Throughout the suturing the nurse, Stephen and Stephen's mother chatted. Much talk was related to Stephen and his school, interposed with explanations as to the next step the doctor was taking in the procedure. 'That is number three, now for number four,' the nurse would say, as the sutures were inserted (local anaesthetic having been used to prevent further pain and distress). On completion Stephen and his mother left the department. What could have been psychologically traumatic turned out to be a simple incident for a happy five year old and a reassured mother.

Coping with Relatives

Helping relatives in times of crisis is another area where nurse intervention is so important. 'I'm sorry Mrs Timms, your husband was dead on arrival.' This sudden news is unfortunately given so often to relatives in the A & E department. Having received a telephone call from well intentioned workmates that Mr Timms had collapsed and been taken to hospital, Mrs Timms arrived expecting to see her husband unwell but not dead. Tears, hysteria, denial, aggression can all be expected from her in this situation. No one can reverse the outcome but nursing intervention does help relatives or friends to adjust to it. It may be that the nurse says nothing but her presence, or perhaps some gesture, will support them and show that she cares. Each situation will be different, each requires a different approach. You should never be left alone in a situation like this, but observing the trained nurse's approach will help you cope with such situations when you are trained. You should observe how the nursing intervention aids distressed relatives and discuss with the trained nurse the type of approach she took and the reasoning behind this.

7 Evaluation

This is the cornerstone to patient care. Unless evaluation takes place, then the goal setting and intervention stages are rather pointless. Evaluation is the means of identifying whether goals have been achieved and if nursing care has improved the situation. In the A & E setting it can determine whether the patient is admitted or discharged home.

Evaluation not only takes place with the patient who presents for the first time, it also takes place on every visit of a patient attending regular follow-up sessions. This re-attendance is normally for redressing of wounds or re-assessment of non-bony injury to limbs. Most of the evaluation is undertaken by nursing staff in the A & E department and if nursing goals have not been met, irrespective of medical goals, the patient may still warrant admission to hospital. For example, the elderly lady who cannot manage at home due to her injury may not require admission on medical grounds but may well need a few days in hospital on nursing grounds.

Some evaluations are quite spectacular and however long you work in A & E, the response of a diabetic patient to glucose or an asthmatic's response to Ventolin nebulisers when suffering an asthmatic attack will still be very dramatic. Also how rewarding it is when, after treatment, a patient can now breathe having arrived with airway obstruction. Nursing intervention is quick: apply suction, position the jaw, place the patient into the recovery position. The goal is to obtain a clear airway. Evaluation finds that a noisy airway full of

Ventolin nebuliser – Ventolin is a broncho-dilator. Given in aerosol form it penetrates into the respiratory tract and improves ventilation.

fluid has changed to a quiet clear airway. Nothing can be more satisfying.

Hypoglycaemia

Diabetes mellitus is a condition where insufficient or total lack of insulin is produced by the islets of Langerhans. The patient thus has a high blood sugar level.

Patients suffering from diabetes mellitus will often be treated with insulin and diet. A number of patients, because of their pace of life, will leave home in the morning having administered their insulin but forgotten breakfast. There is no food to balance the insulin supplied and consequently the blood sugar level falls. The patient may appear drunk, violent, confused or just act very abnormally, sometimes becoming a danger to himself or others. Many patients will suddenly, without warning, fall to the floor unconscious and unresponsive to stimuli. The brain is malfunctioning because of the low blood sugar level.

> ### HISTORY

Steven has been suffering from diabetes since he was twelve. Although his diabetes is well controlled, he tends to rebel slightly towards his disorder. This rebellion has been occurring more frequently as he became older and started wanting to go out and drink with friends of his own age. At least three times a week he overconsumes alcohol and the next morning rejects breakfast while still administering his insulin and this causes some disruption of control.

When Steven becomes hypoglycaemic he is very abusive and has great strength. He seems confused and is unaware of his own body. He talks about his body as if he were detached from it, looking on. When Steven has a normal blood sugar level he is calm, very friendly and all the nurses find him a very kind and caring person.

Assessment and Intervention

Assessment and problem identification pin-point a hypoglycaemic attack. Goals are set:

1 Return blood glucose level to normal.
2 Prevent harm to Steven and staff during his treatment and care.

The action taken is to administer intravenous dextrose. This will increase the blood sugar level and return Steven to his normal calm, friendly state.

Evaluation

1 Have the goals been achieved?
2 Has Steven's blood sugar level returned to normal?

The evaluation is conducted by observations of the signs and symptoms. Steven has become quiet, he is no longer using abusive language. He talks rationally, not imagining himself as being outside his own body. Dextrostix readings indicate blood sugar levels returning to normal.

The fascinating part of this care and treatment is the amount of time involved. The response to treatment is instantaneous. As the dextrose is injected into the vein, the patient's condition changes.

The second goal has also been achieved. Because of adequate staff present and correct handling, neither staff nor Steven have come to harm.

Evaluation has shown that the goals have been achieved, and therefore correct intervention has been carried out. Follow-up by the Diabetic Nursing Officer ensures Steven of full support from the hospital.

Shortness of Breath

Patients presenting with an acute attack of breathlessness on assessment will usually be very anxious, cyanosis may be present and the respiratory rate increased with associated use of accessory muscles. Following medical and nursing intervention an evaluation must be conducted to identify whether goals have been achieved and the problem resolved.

Chronic obstructive airways disease is a condition in which the patient has recurring chest complaints over many years and is thus unable to exchange gases adequately.

Mr Wood, a 75 year old man, had suffered chronic obstructive airways disease for many years. He presented himself at the department suffering from an acute exacerbation. Assessment on arrival indicated cyanosis, generally marked over the face, hands and feet. Respiratory rate was 32 respirations per minute. These were shallow breaths and accessory muscles were in use. Following intervention, goals to improve ventilation, reduce cyanosis and decrease the respiratory rate now required evaluation.

Evaluation

Evaluation indicated a reduced respiratory rate and the respirations had more depth. Tidal volume had thus improved. Cyanosis had decreased, although some cyanosis remained around the lips and earlobes.

Mr Wood was more relaxed and less use was being made of the accessory muscles. The nurse making the evaluation, having compared her findings with the assessment record, could be reassured that intervention had been correct and goals achieved.

Wound Evaluation

Patients who are evaluated on a return visit will be seen more or less frequently depending on the progress of the wound or injury being treated.

Mrs Gilbert had been seen three days ago having sustained a leg injury. She was a 75 year old lady and the wound on her lower leg was a large, very thin tissued laceration. Blood supply to the leg was poor. The wound was holding with the aid of steristrips. The skin flap was cyanosed but appeared viable. A dry non-adherent dressing was applied on top and a support bandage from the base of the toes to just below the knee was used to support the dressing. Mrs Gilbert was seen again three days later; the wound was healing slowly and the skin flap looked much healthier. The dressing was re-applied.

Evaluation

During the evaluation Mrs Gilbert was asked about travelling to and from hospital. As this was proving difficult a community nurse was arranged to call and redress her leg at home. Often a combined care exists between the Accident Department and community nurses, the community nurse being aware of the return visit date (if necessary) and that they can refer back at any time they feel it necessary.

After two weeks Mrs Gilbert was to return for final evaluation; this visit proved beneficial as both nursing and medical staff could see the results of their work. The area on the leg was clean and dry, and the skin flap was of a normal colour. Had the wound become infected, as so many do, and the skin flap necrosed, much more frequent evaluation by both

Necrosis is death of a portion of tissue.

community and hospital care teams would have been required. Dressings would have to have been readjusted in the light of evaluation to meet the altering wound situation.

Summary

Evaluation does not always indicate that intervention has achieved the desired goal, and if so, both goals and action will have to be reassessed and new goals set and action planned. Evaluation is thus a method of periodically determining the patient's response to nursing actions. The time span between evaluations will vary, depending on the condition of the patient and the intervention being undertaken. A patient suffering multiple trauma will require frequent evaluation, possibly every 5 to 15 minutes; patients with other ailments may require half-hourly or hourly evaluation. Other patients may be evaluated in terms of days or weeks.

8 Admission or Discharge

Admission of a patient to hospital is usually based purely on the medical problem. A patient with chest pain may be admitted for observation and further investigation. The same applies to the patient who is suffering acute appendicitis and requires appendicectomy.

On some occasions admission must be based on the person's ability to cope with their injury. For example, an 80 year old woman suffering an arm injury may not be able to cope at home, while a 40 year old person with the same injury may not require admission. In some instances the patient is not suffering from an acute injury or illness but a chronic condition which has become unbearable either for that person or the caring relatives. This situation is often the most difficult to cope with as there is often insufficient reason medically for acute admission but there is a very large social factor. Admission in this type of circumstance usually involves group discussion including nursing staff, social workers, relatives and patient. The decision must ultimately lie with the doctor in charge of the patient but a group discussion makes the decision easier for the doctor.

Whether to discharge or not is usually an easier choice, although again pressure of beds available can often cloud the decision. The majority of patients discharged after examination will fall into three groups:

1   Walking patients who have received treatment for their injury and do not require in-hospital care.
2   Patients who, having come to the department with a potential medical or surgical problem, are either reassured they are not suffering from a particular disorder or given treatment which can be followed up either as an outpatient or by their GP.
3   Self discharge.

Admission

When a decision is made to admit a patient to hospital, the A & E nurse must make preparations for this:
1   Has all treatment given in the A & E department been recorded on the charts?
2   Does the patient understand the need for admission and agree with this course of action?
3   Are the relatives aware of the admission? If present, do they wish to accompany the patient to the ward?
4   Is all property accounted for and checked in to the safe if necessary?
5   What intervention, if any, will be required en route to the ward?
6   Which nurse is best suited to transfer the patient?

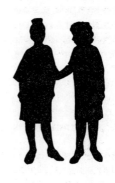

On arrival in the ward the transferring nurse must:
1   Give a full report of the patient's history, treatment and the evaluation made prior to transfer. Has the patient improved?
2   Explain any instruction from the medical staff with regard to continuous treatment, e.g. fluid ratios, drugs to be given.
3   Indicate whereabouts of the relatives, e.g. present or at home, and whether they are aware of the admission.

4   Carry out a property check.
5   Ensure all equipment, pillows, etc. are returned to the A & E department.

Discharge

The vast majority of discharged patients will fall into group 1 (walking patients after treatment). This large group is often the most vulnerable if good discharge advice is not given.

Discharge advice is frequently left to the nursing staff as they usually are the last health care personnel to see the patient. It is essential that, while working in the department, you familiarise yourself with the correct advice to be given to patients on discharge. Generally advice will depend on the particular injury treated, however some points are common to most injuries.

1   How to cope with the dressing, strapping or bandage.
2   When to remove the dressing, strapping or bandage.
3   When to return to their GP or the A & E Follow-up Clinic.
4   What signs and symptoms to watch for while recovering from injury.
5   Has the patient received written instructions on the specific injury, e.g. head injury observation, plaster of Paris check?
6   Has patient been given a letter to inform his GP of the treatment?
7   Has the patient been given a Health Certificate (self certification and, if necessary a Doctor's Certificate)?

Most patients who are sent home have injuries which require care of a dressing and the wound. The care may involve non-bony injury which has been strapped, bony injury supported in a plaster of Paris cast, and post head injury.

Care of Dressing and Wound

Dressings should be kept dry. They should be left in situ unless a specific instruction to remove them or to redress the wound has been given. If the patient is to redress the wound instructions must be given to promote the employment of aseptic techniques. Dressings and equipment must also be supplied. It is pointless to ask a patient to carry out a dressing and then not supply the 'tools' to do the job.

The patient with a sutured wound must be instructed not to pull at the sutures. This especially applies to the scalp where they often can be disturbed by incorrect use of a comb or brush.

Elevation of the limb is important and must be stressed once a wound has been treated.

The patient must be encouraged to return if the wound becomes sore, red or discharges excessively.

Care of the Non-bony Injury

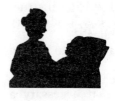

The most common non-bony injury sent home from the A & E department is the sprained ankle. This injury is usually treated with elastoplast strapping or elasticated bandage. Patients must be encouraged to rest the leg in the elevated position. This prevents swelling and allows swelling that has occurred to reduce. Gradually build up mobility to normal within a week to ten days after the injury. The patient must be instructed to observe the toes for good circulation – colour and sensation. Should the strapping become over-tight, it should be removed and the patient return to the department. The strapping should not become wet. Removal is advised after a week to ten days. Cutting the strapping is usually the simplest method of removal. You should always advise the patient that ankle ache may be present for several weeks or months until total recovery is achieved. Slings are used in the treatment of the majority of arm injuries. Patients should be encouraged, if they should not remove the sling, to lift the arm regularly and wash and powder the axilla. Failure to instruct often leads to body odour as the patient is uncertain how much movement is allowed.

Other advice which can be given to patients with an arm injury includes the most comfortable method of dressing and undressing. Always when dressing put the injured arm into the shirt or jumper first. On removal leave the injured arm until last.

Bony Injury supported in a Plaster of Paris Cast

Swelling or incorrect application of POP are two major causes leading to complications for patients. Patients must be instructed clearly and precisely what signs and symptoms to watch for after a cast has been applied.

1 Pain – other than from the injury
2 Colour of toes/fingers – return if cyanosis or pallor develops (circulation impaired)
3 Sensory disturbance in fingers/toes e.g. 'pins and needles', numbness (this can also indicate pressure on nerves)
4 Lack of movement in toes/fingers
5 Swelling of toes/fingers

If any of the above occurs the patient must return immediately.

In addition, the patient must be instructed not to wet the plaster, not to apply force to the cast, and not to push any object down the cast to scratch an itch.

Elevation is again encouraged until the

injury has settled. The patient must be instructed on non-weight bearing or, if allowed to walk, the time from cast application to walking must be delineated.

Post Head Injury

The patient may sleep, but relatives should be encouraged to wake him every hour, then less frequently during the night to assess his conscious level. Instruct the relatives to observe for any vomiting, drowsiness, confusion or continuous crying (in a child). Any concern should be reported to the hospital immediately. No analgesic should be administered for 24 hours because if the headache becomes worse it is an important symptom and should not be masked.

Other common discharge advice involves the correct use of crutches or other aids.

Crutches

Ensure that the crutches are of the correct height for the patient. All patients issued with crutches must be taught the correct method of walking: the crutches are advanced forward, the patient then moves forward, keeping the injured leg from the ground; the leg taking the weight should only come in line with the crutches. Over-swing will throw the person off balance. The importance of returning aids when they are no longer needed must be stressed to each patient, since many departments are constantly having to replace them.

Tetanus Cover

The majority of the community now has received a full course of tetanus prophylaxis. A booster vaccination is usually all that is required. When patients have not received a full course this should be commenced in the A & E department. Follow up injections must be given at 6 weeks' and 6 months' intervals. The patient must be encouraged to receive the next two injections and the staff must explain the necessity of this. (Three vaccinations over a period of 6 months will achieve correct body immunity. Failure to receive the three removes the possibility of adequate cover.)

Antibiotics

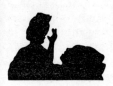

Many patients do not complete a course of antibiotics. You must explain to them that although the symptom of an infection may decrease or disappear, the infective organism will not be totally destroyed if the entire course prescribed is not taken.

Self Discharge

No patient may be held against his will unless a formal restriction is placed as in the case of some psychiatric patients. All patients have the right to refuse treatment and admission to hospital. Nurses should always encourage patients to follow the treatment prescribed and to come into hospital if necessary but they must also respect a patient's wishes. It can be very difficult to understand the reluctance of a person to be admitted and a great deal of tact and diplomacy on the part of the nurse is required. Explanation of possible risk factors must be given.

Any patient who wishes to leave against advice must be referred immediately to a trained member of the nursing staff and to the doctor. If after advice and discussion the patient still wishes to leave, he must be asked to sign a self-discharge form. Treatment should be carried out if the patient agrees and transport home should be arranged if required. Because a patient is taking self-discharge it does not mean that our caring stops.

Discharge Summary

Your patient if discharged leaves your care and undertakes self care of his treated injury. Full explanation and advice must be given. Follow up times or when to return to the GP must be given. Always conclude your discharge care by advising the patient to telephone or return should they be concerned. Remember also patients may need assistance to go home (e.g. if eye pads are used or they have had general anaesthetic always be sure that relatives or friends are contacted if they are not present and will collect the patient).

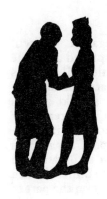

Remember also that patients who are discharged, having come to the A & E department because of a possible medical or surgical problem, are often relieved that their fears have been allayed. The person who thought his chest pain might be cardiac related is a good example. This sufferer will have been very distressed, and being told it is not serious is a great relief to both the patient and his relatives. It is important however that upon discharge the patient must be advised to always seek care should the pain recur. Often the patient, unless encouraged, will not return due to a sense of embarrassment, thinking he has wasted our time on the first occasion. Reassurance and encouragement from nurses do a great deal to remove this embarrassment and reassure the patient.

Conclusion

Most patients are discharged home after treatment. A small percentage of patients are admitted to the hospital. Unless communication and explanation are given, the continuing care of patients will be affected. Remember, just because you know what has happened or what care is required, the ward staff or patient may not. Always be sure that all care given is recorded and information passed on. Self care must be explained fully so that the patient understands. Agreement does not always imply understanding – be sure when you give advice that it is understood. Many departments have printed instruction cards for the patient to follow; these should always be handed out but they must never replace adequate nurse–patient communication.

9 If there is no Acute Medical Problem

Mention was made briefly in the Introduction of patients who arrive in the A & E department without any acute medical problem. Because the department is open twenty-four hours every day, the community expects a service that can cope not only with health but also social needs. In reality the A & E department was not designed to provide such care, but due to closure of many health and social services at the weekends, in the evenings and at night, the public will inevitably arrive at the A & E doors demanding care we cannot always provide.

Medical staff are often unwilling to admit a person simply because they are homeless or unable to cope with the normal functions of daily activity. The nurse within the department can identify more readily through a nursing model the needs of the patient. Unfortunately nurses do not have power of admission and therefore must organise other professions to help in such situations.

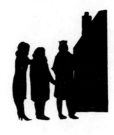

The elderly person who arrives by ambulance on a Saturday afternoon may have many nursing and social needs but no acute medical problem today. The relatives who have coped previously may feel that they can no longer cope with looking after Grandma. The elderly person may have been seen by her GP, who is not available today, and the social worker on call may not be the person who knows this family's problems.

The nurse in the A & E department thus becomes a major part of a care team for this elderly person. There is no acute bed available so a large amount of the nursing care is carried out in the department, while the social services and the family come to a decision. Perhaps the family can be persuaded with extra help to continue their care? Perhaps a short-term bed can be found in an elderly persons' residence? Perhaps an acute geriatric bed is available? There are many possibilities but throughout all the negotiations and discussion the A & E nurse will be involved. Patient care cannot be seen simply as the care of the injured or acutely sick, it must be seen as the response by a nurse to any individual who enters the department, irrespective of others' attitudes. This makes nursing care in A & E different to care provided in any other part of the hospital. The nurse in many of these situations must bring forth all the nursing and social knowledge gained through experience and our unique training.

HISTORY

Mr Smith was well known in the local town. He used to live in a very rundown house before he left the area some months ago. Mr Smith had neglected his general hygiene and appearance but was obviously well educated. Local residents would tell of the sad loss of Mrs Smith many years previously and the general decline in Mr Smith's appearance and care since.

It was just after midnight that Mr Smith was brought into the A & E department. The ambulance crew gave a history of him being knocked over by a car. They had not been able to find any injury but stated that alcohol could be smelt on his breath. When Mr Smith was brought in an assessment was made by the nursing staff.

Assessment

Mr Smith was conscious and orientated to time and place. His clothes were dirty, torn, worn and now wet. The trousers were covered in mud. After helping Mr Smith to undress and put on an examination gown, the nurse undertook a head to toe examination. No injury could be found except a tender area over the right iliac crest and a graze on the right forehead. Mr Smith's hair was dirty and in need of a wash, as was his skin. Oral temperature was 36.5°C, pulse 80, blood pressure 150/80.

The nurse asked Mr Smith what had happened. He gave a history of consuming a few drinks to cheer himself up. As he then did not feel any better, he began to walk. Without looking he started to cross the road and was knocked over. He got up and sat on the verge until the ambulance and police arrived. Mr Smith could give no next of kin or address. He said he left the town some months ago, wandering from area to area, either living in hostels or on the street. Tonight he was going to try and return to his house in this town but then the accident occurred.

Problems

The nurse identified several problems, many of which will require intervention by other professions:

1   Self neglect (actual)
2   Minor injury from accident (actual)
3   Homeless (potential) though Mr Smith's own home would be cold and probably uninhabitable at present
4   Alcohol intake (actual). Inability to look after self?

Goal Setting and Intervention

Short term goals were:

1 To have Mr Smith medically examined. This was undertaken by the Casualty Officer. No injury other than minor bruising to the right iliac crest was found. The abrasion to the forehead required only a clean and antiseptic spray dressing.

2 Provide Mr Smith with a shower and soap. This was undertaken and Mr Smith was able to stand and shower himself. A clean gown and trolley linen were provided.

3 Provide Mr Smith with food and fluid. Although Mr Smith did not feel hungry, he did eat some toast and had a cup of tea.

4 Provide Mr Smith with accommodation. This was a problem. The social worker on call was contacted and the situation presented to her via the telephone.

The Casualty Officer could not justify admission to an acute accident bed as no injury other than an abrasion and bruising was present. Mr Smith was neither dehydrated nor hypothermic.

Although Mr Smith was in need, it was of nursing and social care not of medical care. Nursing care had been provided: his need of body hygiene had been met with the shower, and his need for nutrition and fluid had been satisfied. He was able to cope adequately with all other bodily functions himself. Rest was provided by the use of a patient trolley but no long term residence within the department was possible. To send Mr Smith away from the department to go to his only known home was not acceptable despite the medical discharge.

The outcome of Mr Smith's accommodation crisis in the early hours of the morning will depend very much on the area in which the hospital is situated, the social services available and the accommodation free for such occurrences. Some areas may provide Mr Smith with a short term residence for that morning. Others may only be able to organise such facilities during working hours and Mr Smith may have to remain in the A & E department or the local police station until such arrangements are complete.

Like the elderly person, there is often no easy answer. The nurse must use all nursing skills to provide the patient with the feeling of security and with attention despite the length of arrangements for long term care.

10 Conclusion

There comes a time as a learner when your allocation to Accident & Emergency must come to an end. You will have spent perhaps six or eight weeks within the department and now you can evaluate your time. Have you met your objectives? Remember, these were to learn about conserving life, alleviating suffering and promoting health. Perhaps you were off duty when a patient suffered cardiac arrest or was admitted with multiple injuries, but remember, the one you dealt with complaining of a cut finger, or the mother who had just rushed in with her baby suffering a febrile convulsion, taught you as much, if not more, about individual care.

Upon returning to another ward or the community you may now understand patients in a different way. You now know how acutely ill the man suffering a myocardial infarction was before he arrived on the ward; you also know how distressed his wife and family were when told the news. The young teenage girl who took an overdose of drugs might spend twenty-four hours on the Medical ward; it is much easier for you now to help this individual knowing the immediate care she has had within the A & E unit. If you are continuing your training in the community you will appreciate how important it was to send the patient home from the department with the correct dressings and how frustrating it is if this is not done, or if inadequate information is given.

You will have performed a lot of first aid, admittedly within the department environment, but you can still take this knowledge back to a ward or into the community. You know how not to apply tourniquets, how to apply slings properly and put pressure dressings on wounds. Your practice in care of the person's airway, breathing and circulation puts you in a much better position than before to conserve life.

Do you know more now of the various injuries and illnesses listed in the Introduction? Do you understand better the need for expert nursing care with patients suffering these disorders? Have you acquired some of this expertise? If yes, you have done well; you have achieved your objectives and should feel proud of it.

For those trained nurses who have used this book as a reintroduction to Accident & Emergency nursing, I wish you well in your chosen area of nursing. I encourage you to take hold of all the opportunities available to increase your knowledge and skills in this speciality.

TEST YOURSELF

Finally, I offer you the opportunity of testing your own knowledge with the following questions; the answers are found within the book itself.

1   Mr Reynolds complains of a sore eye. He thinks a piece of dust may have entered the right eye. What assessment would you make of Mr Reynolds?
2   Mrs Jenkins has fallen and injured her elbow. The area is swollen and tender to touch. What assessment and care would you undertake prior to Mrs Jenkins being seen by the doctor?
3   Tim, a seventeen year old student, has been treated for a fractured tibia with a full leg, non-weight bearing plaster of Paris cast. What advice would you give him on discharge from the department?

4   During your assessment of a young man suffering from a chest injury you notice a stab wound with air escaping from the left upper chest. What is your immediate intervention?

5   Mr Stamp arrives in the department complaining of severe central chest pain. He is cyanosed and has a respiratory rate of thirty. Describe your intervention with this man.

6   'Cardiac Arrest five minutes.' This call warns you of a patient's arrival. How do you prepare the resuscitation area of the department for the reception of this person?

7   When assessing a four year old child, what signs would make you suspect that non-accidental injury might be present?

8   Why are Accident & Emergency departments so called?

9   Give some examples of promoting health within A & E.

10 Why should a bandage cover joint to joint?

11 What does the term 'Triage' mean?

12 What is your role in the Triage area?

13 Why is it important to reduce the temperature of a child with pyrexia and hyperpyrexia?

14 If a patient is suspected of suffering a ruptured urethra why should he be asked *not* to pass urine?

15 How would you assess a patient who may be suffering pain but not verbally complaining?

16 What signs and symptoms would make you suspect a patient was suffering obstruction of the blood supply to a limb?

17 List the care, in priority order, for someone suffering multiple injuries.

18 Why should you not carry out full 'lay out' of a person who dies in A & E?

19 How can you best avoid violent situations

developing within the A & E waiting room?

20 Why is it important to determine if a person suffering a head injury has been unconscious at any stage?

21 What potential problems would you anticipate for a patient undergoing a general anaesthetic?

22 Why is it essential to adequately support fractured bones and what methods are available?

23 What signs would make you suspect internal injury of the abdomen, and what intervention would you undertake?

24 What complications can occur when performing a dressing of a burn wound?

25 When admitting a patient to the ward, a number of procedures must be undertaken to ensure smooth transfer of information. List these procedures.

26 Why is tetanus immunity emphasised so greatly in A & E nursing?

27 What instructions should be given to patients when returning home after suturing of a wound has been performed?

FURTHER READING

ASHDOWN, M. 1985. Sudden Death. *Nursing Mirror*, **161**(18):22.

BEDFORD, A. 1985. Child Abuse, the A & E Nurse's Role. *Nursing Mirror*, **161**(16):20.

BRADLEY, D. 1982. *Accident and Emergency Nursing*. London: Baillière Tindall.

BROOKS, E. 1985. Ash Wednesday Disaster. *Nursing Mirror*, **161**(17):30.

FARROW, R. 1964. *The Nursing of Accidents*. London: English Universities Press (Hodder and Stoughton).

HARDY, R. 1976. *Accidents and Emergencies* (Practical Handbook for Personal Use). Oxford: Robert Dugdale.

INTERNATIONAL A/E NURSING CONFERENCE REPORTS. 1985. *Nursing Mirror*, **161**(13,14,15):8.

JOINT AUTHORISED MANUAL OF ST JOHN, RED CROSS. 1982. First Aid Manual. London: Dorling Kindersley Ltd.

MANNING, H. 1985. Sudden Death. *Nursing Mirror*, **160**(18):19.

ROBINSON, J. 1978. *Giving Emergency Care Competently*. Springhouse, Pa:Intermed.

SAFADI, E. 1985. Moving Patients with Head Injuries. *Nursing Mirror*, **161**(6):51.

SYKES, J. 1985. A Night Out on Crutches. *Nursing Times*, **81**(48):32.

TOONEY, S. 1985. Parent's Perception of A/E Care. *Nursing Mirror*, **161**(19):38.

WALSH, M. 1985. *Accident and Emergency Nursing, A new approach*. London: Heinemann.

WRIGHT, B. 1983. Poisoning in Children. *Nursing Mirror*, Oct 19:18.

WRIGHT, B. 1985. Hostility in A/E Departments. *Nursing Mirror*, **161**(14):42.

INDEX